The Practice of
Health Services
Research

The Practice of Health Services Research

Bie Nio Ong

Senior Lecturer and Director
MBA (Health Executive) Programme
Centre for Health Planning and Management
Keele University

CHAPMAN & HALL

London · Glasgow · New York · Tokyo · Melbourne · Madras

Published by Chapman & Hall, 2–6 Boundary Row, London SE1 8HN

Chapman & Hall, 2–6 Boundary Row, London SE1 8HN, UK

Blackie Academic & Professional, Wester Cleddens Road,
Bishopsbriggs, Glasgow G64 2NZ, UK

Chapman & Hall Inc., 29 West 35th Street, New York NY10001, USA

Chapman & Hall Japan, Thomson Publishing Japan, Hirakawacho
Nemoto Building, 6F, 1–7–11 Hirakawa-cho, Chiyoda-ku, Tokyo 102,
Japan

Chapman & Hall Australia, Thomas Nelson Australia, 102 Dodds Street,
South Melbourne, Victoria 3205, Australia

Chapman & Hall India, R. Seshadri, 32 Second Main Road, CIT East,
Madras 600 035, India

Distributed in the USA and Canada by Singular Publishing Group Inc.,
4284 41st Street, San Diego, California 92105

First edition 1993

© 1993 Chapman & Hall

Typeset in 10/12 Palatino by Columns Typesetters of Reading
Printed in Great Britain by Richard Clays Ltd., Bungay

ISBN 0 412 54340 0   1 56593 214 5 (USA)

A catalogue record for this book is available from the British Library

Library of Congress Cataloging-in-Publication data available

For Hilary

Contents

Preface

Writing a book seems a lonely enterprise and I have at times wondered whether it is making me happy. Yet there have been powerful reasons for persevering because this book is a product of much collective thinking, discussion and joint work; it is also the expression of my commitment to improving health and health care through making the process of policy formulation and planning more scientific and democratic. I believe that the development of social science research methods can make a contribution to this process.

The friends and colleagues who have helped me shape my ideas are many. Firstly, Hilary Hodge who set me on this road and gave me the experience at the 'sharp end' of management, but never stifled my thinking and allowed me freedom to experiment and was prepared to take risks. This book is dedicated to her, because of her courage to be an innovative, creative and therefore brave manager. Other colleagues from my time in the NHS are Glenys Marriott, who talked me through many doubts and dilemmas; Gerry Humphris, whose sound scientific approach and rigour saved me from many research disasters, and Sue Jones, who was always enthusiastic in trying out my experiments. Jeff Girling, from the Health Services Management Unit, provided me with a platform for testing out methods and theories. Jeremy Felvus from the Welsh Health Planning Forum read my interpretation of the Welsh strategy.

My colleagues at the Centre for Health Planning and Management, Calum Paton, Mike Rigby and Steve Cropper, gave valuable feedback on my writing; and Chris Shiels did much of the data analysis and kept me on the straight and narrow in quantitative matters. Most importantly, Ken Lee encouraged and supported me throughout my time at the Centre, and urged me to take sabbatical leave in order to write this book. And, of course, Val Watts who protected me from the many possible intrusions on my writing time, and helped to put the manuscript into presentable form.

Furthermore, I have to thank my anonymous referee, who turned out to be David Hunter. He gave me generous and constructive criticism and I have tried to follow his advice. My editor, Rosemary Morris, was always there to help me through hurdles, and demonstrated an unfailing commitment to the project.

Of key importance have been all the people (most commonly called respondents) who have given much of their time and trust to me as a researcher. Many I met in person, and they impressed me with their honesty, the way they coped with misfortune and their willingness to assist with my research, even when I could not promise any direct return for their help. Others I never met, but their contribution to my work has been invaluable.

My home base has been a stable and stimulating environment. Barry Munslow is my most consistent sounding board, and has talked me through the ups and downs of writing, never failing to believe that I could bring this project to a successful conclusion. Karl and Jade continued to put my writing into perspective, and gave me welcome and pleasurable diversions on a daily basis. My parents have showed long-standing and long distance interest.

I cannot say that the production of this book has been a traumatic experience, and the support of those mentioned (and perhaps some who are not mentioned) has helped immeasurably. Of course, the responsibility for the final product rests with myself.

Chapter One

Social science research and health service management

INTRODUCTION

The changes in health policy and strategy in many western developed countries during the 1980s and early 1990s centre around common themes. The economic recession that is gripping Europe and North America and the related political pressures combined with broader uncertainties about the distribution of power and control have caused a major rethinking of the role of welfare. The question of cost containment has floated to the top of the political agenda. Flynn (1992) argues that the key theme for most western developed countries has been the restructuring of state activity in the economy and polity. Many governments have opted to introduce some form of market mechanism in the provision of health care, whether they have a national health service, one based on social insurance or a predominantly private insurance based model.

The question of cost containment in health care has gained more urgency as a result of other pressures bearing on service delivery. The growth in the number of elderly people has been well documented (Jefferys and Thane, 1989) with an expected increase in the use of health services by an ageing population. Furthermore, patterns of social support are changing, which results in people's preference for reliance on formal services rather than the informal sector of care (Daatland, 1989), a trend opposite from the one promulgated by many governments. The dissemination of information about medical advances has been popularized by the media, resulting in a better informed user who demands a fuller range of services, thereby putting pressure on resources. Technical innovations themselves require investment for renewal and update, while not necessarily resulting in medium to long-term cost saving. These combined factors inexorably force the question of cost containment on to health planners and managers.

This context largely determines the research agenda in health which can be defined by either policy makers and managers or by medical professionals, notably public health doctors. There is recognition that the agenda in public health has radically altered and the emergence of the 'new public health' is manifested in changing theoretical approaches (RUHBC, 1989) and research initiatives which bring different disciplines together (Public Health Research and Resource Centre and the University of Salford 1991–1992 seminar series). Yet, more fundamental and widespread developments are needed if health research is to free itself from a medically dominated perspective.

Policy makers and managers have traditionally looked towards medical and clinical research findings, or alternatively, have relied on their own practical knowledge of 'doing the job' of management rather than utilizing the research findings from social scientists. This is in part because the work of social scientists has not been directly related to policy and strategy. Yet, some social scientists have argued that much of their theoretical research has relevance for policy (Stacey, 1991), but in reality only a handful of monographs have been able to influence strategic or managerial decision-making (for example, Cartwright and Anderson, 1982; Townsend and Davidson, 1982; Cox et al., 1987).

Hunter (1990a) puts forward an opposite view when he states that there is a virtual absence of a vigorous health research community, as there is no stable research career structure. Despite the formulation of a national research strategy (Peckham, 1991) in Britain, a top-down dissemination process cannot ensure a change in the culture surrounding research. Hunter argues that managers have to become aware of the possible value of social science research. In turn, researchers have to establish an effective dialogue with managers and communicate their findings in a timely and accessible fashion. The fear amongst social scientists that they will turn into consultants who are mainly deployed to solve problems can be countered by the argument that social science perspectives in themselves have an important contribution to make to health policy and strategy. However, this does mean that involvement in the application of findings in the policy and management field has to be tackled, and social scientists cannot remain aloof.

At the same time, policy makers and managers have to be prepared to adopt a more self-critical stance, and not solely rely on their experiential knowledge based on 'doing'. The reflexivity of the social sciences is an important complement to management handbooks on the one hand, and epidemiological and clinical evidence on the other. For example, one of the key strategies for cost containments has been to extend managerial influence in the health service. Flynn (1992) sets out a framework which places managerial and medical control in an adversarial context, whilst Hunter (1991), in contrast, considers that the key question is how to tackle the management of clinical activity in a way which produces improvement in medical care without alienating the doctors. It is at this interface that the key research questions will be formulated, and where the social sciences can demonstrate their value.

Thus, the main aim of this book is to examine the research agenda as defined by the evolving political context of health services in the developed western world. This agenda conjures up a range of research questions, largely determined by the question of cost containment. The responsibility for resolving this issue lies with managers, who require the co-operation of medical and other health professionals. At the same time research and scientific investigation can provide the underpinnings for managerial decision-making. It is the contribution of social science research to the strategic planning and management enterprise that is the subject of this book.

THE MAIN THEMES

The similarity of the concerns of many western governments brings a series of themes to the surface that have common elements. Despite the differences in the political colour of governments and the differences in health care organizations, the issues for the last decade of this century are all shaped by the combined pressures of advances in health care technology, an ageing population and a contraction of resources for state welfare. Making statements about current and future research themes does not appear to be impossible:

1. Audit and evaluation. In health services research the key concerns are effectiveness, i.e. does the health service achieve its objectives?; efficiency, i.e. the ratio between resource inputs and service outputs (Harrison *et al.*,1990); equity, that is horizontal equity requiring the equal treatment of individuals who are equal in relevant respects, and vertical equity requiring the proportionately unequal treatment of individuals who are unequal in relevant respects (Culyer and Wagstaff, 1992).

2. Needs assessment of populations and individuals, where the concept of need is directly related to the achievement of health gain. This, as a result, encompasses the assessment of needs that can be addressed by the provision of health care, and furthermore, appropriateness and relevance of service provision has to be ascertained. It also encapsulates a contextual understanding of social, economic and cultural conditions and the contribution of other services to the attainment of health. Jefferys (1991) extends this to analysing opportunity and social costs involved in policy and practice options. In a similar manner, Culyer and Wagstaff (1992) state that the identification of resources needed to achieve health is of central concern.

3. User involvement in the planning of services. In order to tailor services to need, the voice of the (potential) users has to be heard both at the level of health policy and strategy, and at the operational level of care provision. The issues of power and control have to be addressed, and the hegemonic power of medical professionals and health managers will be challenged if genuine methodologies to involve users in the decision-making process are adopted. This is not a simple matter, as models of empowerment where technical rather than ideological restructuring has taken place have demonstrated (Hugman, 1991). Research and development of more radical models continues to be an important arena of intellectual activity.

4. Quality of service, that is, to denote how appropriately a particular feature of the care process is carried out (Harrison *et al.*, 1990, p.118) is a theme that carries importance for managers in terms of a cost-effectiveness analysis of what is provided, and for users in relation to the outcome and impact of the treatment received. Quality of life is a more abstract term, located within a specific socio-cultural context. Bowling (1991) discusses the various definitions of quality of life covering a range of components such as functional ability, the degree and quality of social and community interaction, psychological well-being, somatic sensation and life satisfaction. In this volume we will concentrate on the question of who defines quality of life, and focus on the experiential definitions of populations and individuals, rather than on professional measurement of quality of life.

The above themes have been considered by, for example, health economists, geographers, epidemiologists and public health physicians. What then is the distinct contribution of social science research to the analysis of these issues? Social science, and sociology in particular, comprises the study of human social life, groups and societies, and focuses on the subject matter of our own behaviour as social beings (Giddens, 1989). Health, healing and health care structures are legitimate and central concerns for social scientists. Fundamental theoretical work on the concepts of health, illness and sickness as culturally defined forms an essential basis for understanding social actions, including health seeking behaviour and interactions between users and providers of health services. Determinants of health and disease are complex, and the examination of social structures assists in formulating a fuller under-standing of the contextual variables and differences in health between social groupings. Sociological analysis encompasses the historical devel-opment of medical knowledge and professional organization, and it carries out comparative study on institutions and change over time.

The wide ranging analysis afforded by a social science perspective, operating at different levels moving from the individual within a social context to societies at large, allows both an in depth and multifaceted view of health and health care. The methodologies used within the social sciences are consequently wide-ranging and flexible. It is the exploration of when and why these methods can be applied in formulating health policy and strategic management that the following chapters deal with.

THE STRUCTURE OF THE BOOK

Responding to current and future research agendas means a flexible approach to research design. Chapter Two addresses the question of design, that is, making visible the invisible process of targeting research methodologies to the questions under examination. Designing research involves a series of choices, weighing up the strengths and weaknesses of different methods in relation to the aims and objectives of research. The collaboration between researchers and those who use the findings (and sometimes these are the same people) is essential if social research is to show relevance for decision-making in policy and planning.

Chapter Three discusses the place of surveys in health policy research by delineating the scope and purpose of the method, and its costs and benefits. The propensity of health service managers to choose the survey as their preferred option will be scrutinized, because it is often related to an incomplete and sometimes misguided understanding of the outcomes of a survey. There are ample examples of good health survey research, but the lessons offered by these examples have to be studied carefully before the method is adopted for planning purposes. An adaptation of the Cambridge Health and Lifestyle survey (Cox *et al.*, 1987) in one health district will serve as an illustration of the method and the type of results that are generated.

Harrison *et al.* (1990) state that the history of evaluation in the British health service is very short indeed, and that up to the 1980s little systematic evaluation of the extent of cure or care or improvement took place. This picture is not very dissimilar to that in other developed western health care systems, but by the 1980s evaluation had become a necessary and accepted instrument in health services management.

Numerous methods of evaluation have been developed, and it is beyond the scope of the discussion in Chapter Four to review all of them. Instead, the argument will be put forward that evaluation has to be an integral part of the management process and closely linked to the setting of aims and objectives. Thus, evaluation can be utilized in different ways, either to refine and adjust objective setting, or to judge the 'value' of particular interventions. Both types of evaluation are illustrated in Chapter Four by detailing two projects, one evaluating the organizational impact of new medical technology, the other to assess the quality of life of people discharged from long-stay mental institutions.

Chapter Five focuses on a method which is considered as a quintessential anthropological approach, namely ethnography. This chapter intends to demonstrate the relevance of ethnographic research for managerial decision-making. The essence of ethnography is that it attempts to theoretically describe social realities through the production of concepts and models that allow people to see events in new ways. The description takes place within context, thus trying to capture the totality or 'richness' of what the social situation presents. This multilayered and dense analytical approach is topical for strategic management which is geared to cultural change. The description of organizational processes, perceptions and ways of thinking of actors within organizations is of immense value for understanding the internal workings of social structures. The study by Strong and Robinson (1990) provides powerful insights into how the 1983 changes in the British NHS have been interpreted throughout the service.

In this chapter a similar example will be discussed demonstrating the application of ethnography within the management of change, while the second example focuses on understanding the experience of illness and nursing care. This study was designed to develop concepts and indicators for assessing district nursing, and applied ethnographic interview methods in order to uncover the perceptions of users and carers.

Chapter Six deals with two key issues in health policy, namely the assessment of need and user participation. It discusses a methodology grounded in the tradition of action research and community development, which combines the formulation of priority need with involving (potential) users in the planning of services. This method is still evolving, which makes it particularly interesting from a methodological point of view, because it offers a greater degree of flexibility in dovetailing the research with the policy and strategy process.

Whilst the first six chapters focused on particular methodologies, the implicit assumption has been that there is no single best methodological answer to the infinitely complex problems faced in health and health care. Chapter Seven takes this challenge on board and discusses the increasingly accepted option of designing multimethod research. Having examined the strengths and weaknesses of various social science methods it seems logical to create a methodological 'jigsaw' which is capable of balancing different approaches in a way which allows the optimal and most penetrating analysis of strategic issues. The examples given in this chapter are concerned with two central questions in the western world, namely the needs of the elderly population, and multi-organizational responses to the delivery of care for specific client groups, in this case, people with physical disabilities.

The final chapter of this book reiterates the argument that the common problems faced by health services in developed countries require a concerted effort across various disciplines, including the social sciences. The specific contribution of social science lies in its capacity to examine social structures, behaviours and ways of thinking, and the methodologies employed are varied and flexible. The important question is to design research in ways that fully exploit the methodological possibilities offered by the social sciences in order to provide a theoretically grounded framework for health policy and strategy.

Chapter Two

Choices in social science research design

INTRODUCTION

Social scientists have traditionally made distinctions between theoretical research, policy oriented and applied research. Broadly, the concern of theoretical or 'pure' research is with the advancement of knowledge, and tends to be unidisciplinary. It primarily seeks legitimation from the academic community. Policy oriented research is directed towards outcomes, and reflects organizational aims and objectives. Here, research is perceived as action, to assist informed decision-making, implementation and evaluation. Its main audience are the policy makers, those who take decisions at strategic levels and other similar groupings. Applied research is theoretically based, but oriented to specific problems which can be research driven or instigated by policy makers. It has the purpose of extending knowledge in one particular area of social problematic, and as a result appeals to both academics and policy makers.

Hunter (1990b) observes that social science research has hardly contributed to the changes in health policy in the last decade and a half. Yet, it could be argued that health research has to operate within the policy field, at local or national levels. The difference in locus affects the scope and depth of the research undertaken, while the subject matter of health and health related issues remains the same. The evidence that health is not a unitary but a multidimensional concept is well established (Blaxter, 1990), and consequently, health research has to be multidimensional and multidisciplinary. Policy oriented research has the same propensity in its search to form a fully rounded and balanced picture on any topic (Hakim, 1987). Based on this similarity the chapter will develop its argument that the question of research design has to be central. As a result the theoretical divide between quantitative and qualitative research will be largely demystified, and limited to a technical distinction. I will argue that in order to contribute to understanding the complexities of the health experience, and the variety of policy and service responses, researchers have to choose from a range of possible methodologies, and cast aside entrenched theoretical or ideological positions. Instead, attention has to be concentrated on creating research designs which are capable of tackling the important health problems of our time by drawing on the most effective and efficient combination of scientific methods.

DESIGNING RESEARCH

The majority of research textbooks deal with how to do research, that is, with the methods, techniques and operational details. Often, a brief discussion on the theoretical underpinnings of particular methodologies is presented. Increasingly, researchers are becoming aware that design questions, namely when and why particular approaches are selected, have to be explicitly addressed (Hakim, 1987). Professional researchers do make design choices, but do not tend to describe these explicitly. Justifying a particular design is becoming more common with funders inquiring about the cost-effectiveness of specific methodologies in achieving intended outcomes. This is an important development, not only for demystifying the research activity, but also in making visible the invisible work of creating research. In doing so, others can learn from seeing how problems have been translated into researchable questions, and understand the crucial role of design. Thus, in Hakim's words, design deals primarily with aims, uses, purposes, intentions and plans within the practical constraints of location, time, money and availability of staff (Hakim, 1987, p.1).

By defining research design as being firmly located in the real world, the range of choices to be made is related to key issues such as setting clear aims and objectives which focus on policy questions and sharpen the research exercise. It also draws researchers into the arena of outcomes, which can demand accountability for research findings and applications. Collaboration with the people one does research for or on is an important concern, and the financial management of research activities is an integral part of the total process. This means that researchers have to assess the choices available to them within the policy and strategy context, which forces them to place the question of design centre stage, as they will be held accountable for the process and outcome of research.

Research design is not only the prerogative of researchers, even though their theoretical and technical expertise plays a crucial role. It is as much a political question where the sponsors want to set the agenda. They have specific purposes and intended outcomes in mind, and the process of doing research can be significant in their goal attainment. For example, in carrying out user feedback research multiple aims can be formulated, incorporating measuring the quality of service in order to market a 'product', assessing clinical practice or focusing on health gain. These different goals are not mutually exclusive, and can be pursued alongside each other, either implicitly or explicitly. Yet, the researcher has to be aware of the range and the nature of the various goals in order to design and control the research effectively.

This is not an easy task because agreement on aims, purpose and use of research is the result of negotiation between researchers, sponsors and participants. Apart from these fundamental questions the operational aspects of research have to be resolved, and often depend on agreement about principles. I have argued elsewhere (Ong, 1989) that this places the researcher in a methodological and political conundrum. The problem is not just one of 'handing over' the research findings to policy makers and managers, which some have argued helps to maintain the status quo (Wenger, 1987). Setting objectives with sponsors is a double-edged sword: on the one hand access to research sites is facilitated, confidence about implementation of findings and influencing change is increased; on the other hand, certain groups will automatically distrust the researcher, precisely because of the connection with sponsors, and the researcher's ability to develop a critical and rounded analysis can be seriously hampered.

The implications are that the design process becomes more visible, but with it also the role of the researcher. In policy oriented research this role can be variously defined: it can mirror the anthropological self, where the researcher is an insider (Whyte, 1984); it can take the form of advocacy (Salmen, 1987); it can be an agent of change (Lees and Smith, 1977) or in contrast, the researcher can be the outsider looking in and examining the development and implementation of policy (Pettigrew *et al.*, 1988; Flynn, 1992). There is considerable argument as to which approach has most chance of influencing policy. Hunter (1990c) points out that much social science research challenges cherished assumptions and appears de-stabilizing, and therefore is not welcomed by policy makers. However, this does raise the question as to how researchers should relate to the people who formulate policy and strategy in order to come to a closer 'fit' between research and the direction of policy and planning.

This brings us back to the issue of agreeing the aims and objectives of research. Sponsors have to be clear about their own purpose, and understand the specific contribution that research can make in its achievement. Researchers need a similar clarity about their purpose, the researchability of the problem under consideration and the definition of their own role. Only then can discussions about an appropriate research design take place as the political and theoretical considerations are setting the conceptual framework for making decisions about methodologies and techniques.

QUALITATIVE AND QUANTITATIVE RESEARCH

Scientific debate about the relative merits of quantitative versus qualitative methods has influenced the perceptions of the people who commission or use social science research. Stereotypical ideas of quantitative research as presenting hard data, being objective, scientific, structured, reliable and hypothesis testing are contrasted with qualitative research offering soft data, being subjective, pre-scientific, unstructured, rich and illustrative (Halfpenny, 1979; Bryman, 1988). Whatever adjectives are used, most observers see the two approaches as diametrically opposed, and this is very marked within the health sector. There, the dominance of medico-scientific research sets the parameters for all other research and determines which paradigm is deemed bona fide. This tendency leads to label surveys, experimental designs or longitudinal studies as accepted types of study.

The dichotomy leads to misunderstanding of the strengths and weaknesses of the different methods, and narrows the range of choices for good research design. However, there is no 'absolute' qualitative or quantitative approach, in that each is inextricably related to theoretical perspectives employed within a study. For example, positivists aim to establish causal connections between variables, that is to establish laws, and link these laws into deductively integrated theory. For them quantitative data is expressed in mathematical or formal language, while qualitative data is expressed in natural or informal language. This can be compared with the interpretivists, who search for cultural meaning and who intend to establish patterns of interaction which are understandable within a particular culture. They consider quantitative data as marginal to their enterprise because this type of data is not capable of uncovering the subjective meaningfulness that qualitative data can offer (Halfpenny, 1979). In short, what is considered qualitative or quantitative depends on the theoretical approach adopted.

It could be argued that the quantitative–qualitative divide is a smokescreen, because in reality researchers do not adopt 'pure' methods. Many qualitative studies use quantitative concepts when they, for example, state 'a few respondents felt' or 'the majority of people interviewed said'. Conversely, quantitative studies attempt to assign meaning. Finch (1987) discusses the vignette technique in survey research, which is a method that invites respondents to make normative statements about a set of social circumstances. The technique acknowledges that meanings are social and that morality may well be situationally specific. Employing this method within quantitative research enriches the findings, rather than contaminating its methodological purity.

Bryman (1988) insists that 'the distinction between quantitative and qualitative research is really a technical matter, whereby the choice between them is to do with their suitability in answering particular research questions' (p.109). To take this further, placing quantitative and qualitative data in two separate categories can be considered fallacious, and it will be more productive to see them on a continuum ranging from more to less precise data (Hammersley, 1992).

Hammersley (1992) elaborates on further apparent distinctions between qualitative and quantitative approaches, and argues that it should not be the case that the opposition of models is at issue, but that a range of positions is possible, sometimes located on more than one dimension. He does not see the adoption of positions as mutually exclusive, but emphasizes that selection of a particular position depends more on the purposes and circumstances of research than on being derived from methodological and philosophical commitments. He argues that researchers are constantly engaged in trade-offs, and constantly face choices in research. The qualitative–quantitative divide reduces the view and obscures the complexity of the problems that the world presents. Instead, opening up the range of methodological choices assists in making effective design decisions and focuses the research enterprise.

This position is well summarized by Bryman (1988) when he states that 'there should be a greater recognition in discussions of the general aspects of social research methodology of the need to generate good research. This injunction means attending to the full complexity of the social world such that methods are chosen in relation to the research problems posed' (p.173).

The value of the broader perspective on methodologies is demonstrated in health service research. Popay *et al.* (1992) argue that in the field of health needs assessment the full range of quantitative and qualitative approaches can be employed, and discuss in depth the respective strengths and weaknesses in order to build up a design which consists of complementary methods allowing a complex picture to emerge. It is important to distinguish different objectives within the research: for example, if you want to know how many people smoke, a quantitative study can provide the answers; if you want to know why people smoke, a qualitative study will be more suitable.

In conclusion, research design decisions are determined by theoretical, methodological and political factors. This requires that researchers are first of all concerned with setting clear objectives with sponsors in order to determine the framework which will guide research choices. The dichotomy between quantitative and qualitative approaches is not considered helpful; instead a more flexible and pragmatic approach is taken whereby the purpose and context of research direct the way in which complex problems are to be examined. In health services research this appears to be an appropriate stance, precisely because the type of problems encountered in the health field tend to be multidimensional, and as such call for a research approach drawing on a broad spectrum of methodologies which can be integrated (Whyte, 1984).

HEALTH POLICY AND STRATEGY

The World Health Organization set an important example with the formulation of a strategy for health with its 'Health for All by the Year 2000' approach (WHO, 1981 and 1985). Enthusiasm for this strategic approach has been variable across the world, and Britain has been slow in taking it up. Rathwell (1992) reviews the British response and provides several explanations for this reluctance, such as the unresolved debate around inequalities in health, the reorganizations in the health service itself and the lack of clarity about the role of Public Health. The two areas in which a strategic approach has been most consistently – if not unproblematically – adopted are health promotion (Farrant, 1991) and the 'Healthy Cities Project' (Ashton, 1992). Only in 1991 did the Government publish its first consultative document on a national health strategy (DoH, 1991a) with the publication of the final strategy in July 1992 (DoH, 1992). The strategy defines an overall health gain direction and sets five key target areas. The strategy is firmly linked with the overall health reforms and the national research and development strategy plays an important role in delivering on the targets. It is too early to judge the success of the national strategy, but important theoretical (and political) weaknesses have been pointed out, most notably the reluctance to accept the link between poverty and ill health as a fundamental basis for inequalities in health (Limb, 1992). This poses questions as to what parameters for strategic research will be set and the extent to which research findings can alter target setting, and how these targets are to be achieved.

Wales was the first country in the United Kingdom that formulated a Strategic Intent and Direction for its health service (Welsh Office, 1989a) and a concomitant planning framework (Welsh Office, 1989b). The two documents define a strategic direction which contains three elements:

- health gain focused: the NHS in Wales seeks to add years to life through a reduction in premature deaths and life to years through improvement in well-being for both patients and the population at large;
- people centred: the NHS in Wales should value people as individuals and manage its services to this end;
- resource effective: the NHS in Wales should strive to achieve the most cost-effective balance in its use of available resources (Welsh Office, 1989a, p.7).

This leads to the formulation of a strategic intent: 'working with others, the NHS should aim to take the people of Wales into the 21st century with a level of health on course to compare with the best in Europe'.

The Strategic Intent and Direction (SID) is operationalized into a planning framework based on key features such as a structure which links strategy and direction at the all-Wales and local levels; with a primary focus on identifying opportunities for health gain; a recognition that the development of effective strategies depends on an assessment of the needs of local people and communities; the active involvement of all key parties in the strategy formulation process and so on (Welsh Office, 1989b, p.9).

The planning framework has a District focus, but at the same time an overall direction has to be maintained in the development of local strategies for the ten specified Health Gain areas. These areas have been nationally determined as follows: maternal and early child health, cardiovascular diseases, cancers, physical disability and discomfort, respiratory disease, injuries, emotional health and relationships, mental distress and illness, healthy environments, mental handicap. Protocols have been developed for some of the areas (for example cancers, respiratory disease, maternal and child health, physical disability and discomfort) with the intention to cover all other areas in a similar way. Each protocol identifies where further investments could bring worthwhile health gain, and it indicates where current practices are questionable and reinvestments might be considered.

A clear overall strategic framework has been defined in Wales, which delineates the agenda for policy research. It can be best illustrated when considering the development of local strategies, which firstly have to be based on assessing the needs of general populations, specific client groups, and sometimes of individuals. There is no established science of needs assessment, but the SID emphasis on health gain and people centredness determines the nature and form of needs assessment. An important basis is epidemiological research which is capable of providing a longer term perspective on trends in mortality and morbidity, and thus offers historical comparisons, but also comparisons with other countries. All the protocols use this type of research.

Research on inequalities in health is an important element in comparing trends among different social groupings in society. Whilst general mortality has improved in the UK, social disparities continue to exist, and in some cases are widening (Jacobson *et al.*, 1991). This type of research has to stray into a variety of areas, including socio-economic aspects, occupational health, environment, professional and political decision-making, lifestyle and behaviour. The latter two elements have tended to be overemphasized, with the danger of attributing individual responsibility to health. The choices in behaviour, however, have to be contextualized as social, environmental and economic circumstances are important determinants.

When operationalizing the people centredness theme, health beliefs have to be examined. Social scientists have emphasized the importance of the distinction between disease and illness, whereby disease is understood as a malfunctioning of the body expressed in clinical categories, whilst illness is seen as the experience of disorder framed by cultural categories. Therefore, research on the needs of populations and individuals has to understand the illness experience, and then include an understanding of health beliefs of different socio-cultural groupings. Perceptions of the needs for health care are similarly culturally circumscribed. Participation by (potential) users in determining a needs profile becomes essential if the cultural notions are to complement the epidemiological data bases.

Turning to health care provision itself, questions about its aims and objectives have to be guided by the needs assessment, whilst critically examining current practice. This means analysing patterns of service provision and their underlying rationales, in particular the ways in which services contribute to achieving health gain. Furthermore, the people centred focus draws attention to the development and application of user feedback research. This encompasses both user satisfaction, and a wider evaluation of how the content and nature of service provision are responsive to user need. For example, service uptake figures have to be complemented by research into the reasons why people do not take up certain services.

The outcome and impact of services have to be researched, in particular their contribution to the short, medium and long-term quality of life of individuals. This is, as yet, an uncertain science, but models are being developed which contribute to an understanding of the theme 'adding life to years'. A variety of measurement tools exists (Bowling, 1991; Wilkin *et al.*, 1992), which can suitably form part of an experimental or before–after study design. In addition, more qualitative and context specific studies have been carried out, for example on obstetric care (Oakley, 1981a; Porter and MacIntyre, 1984), which provide insight into the experience of receiving health services and their impact on quality of life.

The formulation of local strategies requires an assessment of response options in order to select preferred options which will direct the purchasing actions. Jacobson *et al.*, (1991) argue that broadly two public health approaches exist:

- the 'population approach' which focuses on measures to improve health throughout the community (original emphasis);

- the 'high risk' approach which concentrates action on those who are at highest risk of ill health (p.14).

Alongside these two groupings, actual service patterns have to be studied and compared with alternative modalities of care. Despite the difference in focus, all three approaches require evaluation.

First, equity is an issue whereby the population approach is tested on whether it can achieve a more equal distribution of health among the population. When selecting the risk approach, will a targeted distribution of resources achieve equity in health, or deprive other groupings of necessary services? Furthermore, have alternative options been explored or developed which are better at achieving equity, and address priority needs?

Second, when employing the population approach, accessibility has to be ascertained, and research can explore barriers to service uptake. This is even more important when targeting risk groupings, which can be diffuse, who resist intervention or who are difficult to define. Exploratory research is capable of addressing some of these issues, demarcating the areas for attention and setting out the parameters for action. Similarly, when weighing up alternatives accessibility for each option has to be explored.

Third, acceptability falls within the people centredness arena, where dialogue with users about the various types of service provision is essential. Using the population approach perceptions of communities about priorities will guide intervention strategies. When opting for the risk approach, more in-depth assessment of specific subgroupings has to be made in order to gauge their attitudes and understanding of targeted services. It is important that social groups are not 'labelled', if their co-operation is sought. Community development or action research approaches are possible methods within this context.

Finally, resource effectiveness is a central concept in the Welsh strategy. This is a rapidly developing area of research, of which cost effectiveness analysis and future scenario development are the two most visible branches. Considering the first approach it is important to make a distinction with cost-benefit analysis, where the issue to be evaluated is whether a service should be provided, and which involves attempting to place a value on the quality of life, or changes in it, for those people who receive the service (Davies, 1987). Costs and benefits are valued in commensurate terms, usually money, so that one benefit may be directly offset against the other (Shiell and Wright, 1990). There are, however, obvious difficulties of valuing health care benefits in those terms.

Cost effectiveness analysis asks the question 'what is the best method of giving such a service?'. It can either assume that the outcomes of each alternative are the same in quality of life terms and then evaluate which costs the least, or that the outcome of each option is different and give an implied cost per unit (Davies, 1987). However, the reality is often infinitely more complex, and alternative health care programmes do not have the same effect, or have a variety of benefits along different dimensions. A very important consideration is the time horizon taken for an evaluation, whereby particular investments can be cost-effective if a sufficiently long time span is taken, but not show up over short time lags. In effect, cost effectiveness analysis requires a range of sophisticated methods and tools, often beyond the scope of the average health strategist or manager. This means that research expertise in certain key areas has to be brought in from outside, and in close collaboration with managers and service providers, methods have to be tested and refined.

The field of futures research in health is expanding, and some governments have noted the relevance of this work for their own policy formulation (notably the Netherlands). Futurism is defined as constructively thinking about the future, and trying to anticipate the range of potential events or conditions. It enables people, on the one hand, to prepare for them and, on the other hand, to make some informed choices about them. Futurism is concerned with medium to long-term (5–20 years or longer) predictions within the context of plausibility. An important role for futurism is to create images of preferable futures, but to leave it to decision-makers to influence the direction of their own preferred future (Bezold. *et al.*, 1991).

The research design used by the STG in the Netherlands (Steering Committee on Future Health Scenarios, 1991) consists of three elements:

1. The current scale of the problem under study (for example, diabetes mellitus) is examined and an analysis made, where possible, of the trends in the recent past.
2. A list of possible futures is drawn up, often done with the aid of a Delphi study. This can be done by distributing questionnaires to a number of experts in the field and discussing the results in a workshop, in order to achieve a level of consensus.
3. A number of scenarios are then drawn up which differ in terms of assumed 'autonomous' developments, and the scope for influencing these developments through government action or by other social groupings. The implications of the various scenarios at a specific point in the future can then be calculated with the aid of a computer model.

This approach offers the possibility of changing strategy and planning from being based on an assessment of past successes and failures to attempting to shape the future by deliberately modelling it through calculated choices. The orientation of deciding preferred options moves from a concern with the present to one that deals with present and medium to longer term future. The interplay between policy, strategy and research is essential in this field, and constant feedback loops have to be built in if the overall strategy is to provide the conceptual framework.

In Wales both cost-effectiveness analysis and future scenario research are employed in the development and implementation of the strategy. For example, research and a conference examining the future of the hospitals (Banta, 1990) have stimulated thinking across the service, and informed planning strategies. The continuing dialogue between researchers and policy makers is a central element in the Welsh approach, and pushes back the boundaries of both the research and management enterprises.

CONCLUSION

Social scientists have an important contribution to make to health policy and strategy, but can only do that if they are in direct communication with the people who define them. At the same time, research fulfils its potential within a clearly defined context, and the discussion of the Welsh situation demonstrates that research guided by an explicit strategic direction is capable of defining its objectives and outcomes. More importantly, the discussion has emphasized the centrality of research design, which allows researchers to make explicit choices about methodologies and purpose within given constraints, and be accountable for the choices they make.

Thus, the debate about qualitative versus quantitative research becomes obsolete, and moves instead into the arena of when and why to apply a particular method for addressing a particular question. This is important in health research, precisely because health and health care are multidimensional and complex concepts, which require a multimethod approach. This is illustrated when discussing the Welsh model, whereby three key themes underlie the total policy and planning process, demanding a flexible and layered design model.

This book will continue to emphasize this flexibility when reviewing the different social science methods and their applications. Few of the chosen methods are the only alternative to analysing specific problems, but have been incorporated in the particular research designs, given the context (time, place, people, money, skills, constraints, etc.) in which the work is carried out. The fact that social scientists have a range of methods at their disposal, and can utilize them with a large degree of creativity and flexibility, constitutes their attractiveness for policy makers and managers. They can learn these methods themselves, or (as knowledgeable contractors) employ social researchers. The resulting dialogue about appropriate research designs will strengthen and deepen the process of health policy and strategy.

Chapter Three

Surveys in health services research

INTRODUCTION

Survey research has been an accepted and established part of health research, and a comprehensive review carried out by Cartwright (1983) demonstrates the scope of surveys and the variety of methods employed within this field. Most of the surveys she reviews, however, are relatively large undertakings, either because they are part of a national study, such as the General Household Survey, or because they are separately funded academic pieces of work. On the whole, surveys to assist local decision-making processes have to be more modestly designed.

The potential of surveys is increasingly being recognized by policy makers and managers, but they often have a limited understanding of the relative strengths and weaknesses of the approach. On the other hand only a minority of academic researchers have experience of carrying out survey research specifically tailored to health care decision-making, leaving much of this terrain to market researchers or social research organizations.

It is important, though, for social scientists to operate within the field of health survey research in order to demonstrate the link between social research and theory. De Vaus (1990) argues that theory development and theory testing are important goals for social research and, by extension, for survey research, because researchers are trying to understand *what* is going on and *why* it is going on (p.11, original emphasis). In so doing the concepts used for policy and strategic management can be developed on the basis of scientific evidence, enriching the frameworks employed by health professionals. This would counterbalance the uncritical reliance on inadequate studies carried out in the health service under the label of 'survey'.

This chapter, therefore, will start off with defining surveys, their application and strengths and weaknesses, before outlining the skills and resources required for survey research. Two examples of recent surveys specifically commissioned for strategic planning of health services will be discussed. The first one is a district-based survey modelled on the national Health and Lifestyle Survey (Cox. *et al.*, 1987); the second, a user feedback survey on selected Regional Specialties, aimed at developing a tool to be used for a range of other specialties.

THE SURVEY METHOD

There are numerous standard texts explaining the principles and practice of the survey methodology (for example, Hyman, 1955; Moser and Kalton, 1971; Hoinville *et.al.*, 1977; de Vaus, 1990), and we refer for scientific guidance to any of these volumes. Instead, this chapter briefly discusses the definitions of the survey method, and its relevance for the health field.

Marsh (1982) offers an important assessment of the contribution of surveys to sociological explanation, and defines the survey as follows:

- Systematic measurements are made over a series of cases yielding a rectangle of data.
- The variables in the matrix are analysed to see if they show any patterns.
- The subject matter is social (p.6).

De Vaus elaborates on this definition by stating that 'surveys are characterized by a structured or systematic set of data which I will call a variable by case data matrix. All it means is that we collect information about the same variables or characteristics from at least two (normally far more) cases and end up with a data matrix. In other words, for each case we obtain its attribute on each variable. Put together we end up with a structured or "rectangular" set of data' (p.4–5).

In relation to the scope of surveys Cartwright says that 'surveys are essentially a research tool by which facts can be ascertained, theories confirmed or refuted, ideas explored and values identified and illuminated. So the sorts of questions with which the surveys are concerned relate to the distribution and association of facts and attitudes' (Cartwright, 1983, p.1). Kerlinger (1973) specifies the interests of the survey researcher as examining sociological facts, which are attributes that spring from their membership in social groups, for example income, political persuasion or education; and psychological facts, which include opinions and attitudes. In short, the survey researcher wants to know what people think and what they do.

In order to interpret these two types of facts, the survey researcher has to build a causal model which looks at various kinds of possible relationships between variables. Hellevik (1984) argues that 'models may be classified as general or specific depending upon whether the assumptions made are restricted to what variables to include in the model and how to order them, or in addition specifications with regard to the sign or size of effects are made' (p.52). Therefore, models vary greatly in complexity and explanatory power, and require a considerable amount of expertise in quantitative data analysis.

At this point, it is relevant to turn to Marsh's discussion on the application of the survey as distinct from an opinion poll. She argues that, scientific sophistication aside, the ideal type of survey is performed to better understand something, while a poll tends to be part of a democratic process, that is, people's views have to be recorded in order to give a fair picture of what people think. Marsh stresses that any particular piece of research is likely to have elements of each ideal type (p.126), but the distinction is important, considering that much health policy research is targeted at eliciting opinions of users in order to decide on the nature and scope of service provisions.

In terms of data analysis the opinions and attitudes expressed in surveys are treated as variables for building models to explain clusters and structures in value systems, while in polls they are seen as equivalent to 'votes'; for example, 70% of respondents think that outpatient appointment systems are satisfactory, and therefore it is concluded that no change is needed. This does not, however, analyse the rationales behind giving such answers, which could reflect a sense of powerlessness to change systems or of having low expectations. Yet, many politicians and managers use survey results as if they were poll results, therefore overlooking the meaning behind the results and thus failing to uncover possible discrepancies between what people say and what they do. It is precisely this type of inconsistency that researchers find interesting (Marsh, 1982) and the first case example will demonstrate this.

HEALTH SURVEYS

Cartwright (1983) relies in her review of health surveys on the definition given by Platt, which contains as its main elements systematic and structured questioning (about attitudes, opinions and behaviour) and targeting a relatively large number of respondents. The key methodological problem is the task to measure the subjective aspects of people's meanings and intentions. One important issue is the often committed fault of inferring causality from correlation. It is, therefore, essential that sample size must be large enough to ensure adequate representation of cases in the analytical subcells (Marsh, 1982). Thus, in planning health surveys the research aim has to be clearly delineated in order to justify the choice of the survey approach, both on methodological and cost-effectiveness grounds.

The choice of the survey as the preferred method should first and foremost be on the grounds that it suits the research problem (de Vaus,

1990) which, of course, is the case with choosing any methodology. Cartwright's review (1983) presents the range of subjects suitable for applying the survey method in the health field, including the use of general measures of health and sickness to make comparisons over time; understanding the nature of disease by, for example, uncovering causality or identifying syndromes; assessing health and health care needs of populations; evaluating the use of services; examining the effects and side effects of care; studying the acceptability of services or investigating the organization of care.

The above list includes both regular surveys, such as the health related questions in the General Household Survey, and ad hoc sample surveys, such as Blaxter's study of the meaning of disability (1976). Hakim argues that ad hoc sample surveys have many advantages: first, the application of sampling allows the production of descriptive statistics that are representative of the whole study population, but at a much lower cost than with a census of every member of the population in question; second, they allow associations between factors to be mapped and measured; third, they can be used to study causal processes; fourth, they are increasingly used to complement and extend the information from regular surveys by more detailed investigation of particular topics or populations. Furthermore, the sample survey design is attractive to policy makers because of its *transparency* or *accountability*; that is, the fact that the methods and procedures used can be made visible and accessible to other parties, so that the implementation and the overall research design can be assessed (Hakim, 1976, p.48, original emphasis). By the same token, it lays the survey method more open to criticism, and both Marsh (1982) and de Vaus (1990) deal extensively with the different critiques, including philosophical and methodological attacks.

In *The Natural History of a Survey* Cartwright and Seale (1990) provide an insightful and detailed account of the methodological, ethical and operational issues involved in carrying out a large survey. This is an extremely informative piece of work for new and experienced survey researchers alike, as it offers a frank narrative of the problems and joys of research. It is particularly relevant for the health context because of its subject matter, namely life before death, focusing on all aspects of terminal care. The role of the researcher, not just as a technical expert but very much as a social persona, able to convince funders, ethical committees, respondents and co-workers of the relevance and importance of the study aims and methods, emerges powerfully. The survey researcher as a manager of people and of other resources is emphasized throughout.

At the same time, the book offers a good blueprint for the different stages of survey research in health settings. It discusses the total process from inception, the pilot, sampling frame, ethical approval, interviewing the various subsamples, data preparation and analysis to the presentation of the results. Interestingly, it also discusses the training of interview personnel, and their own evaluation of the training and the project as a whole. The design of this study merits the attention of everyone embarking on health survey research.

One issue that is increasingly addressed by researchers and those commissioning research is the cost of survey research. It is an accepted fact that surveys are expensive, because of their size and complexity. The question of whether the original problem and the expected research outcomes warrant the cost has to be answered at the outset. Certain authors address these practical aspects of surveys particularly well, offering a range of alternatives with varying resource implications (for example, Hoinville *et al.*, 1977). Choices can be made about sample size and type, interview procedures, data sources and analyses, each of which have different implications for the composition of the research team and the financial and computing resources needed. Hakim (1987) argues that researchers and managers can always explore the possibility of 'trading down' to a less expensive – and often different – research design, without major compromises as to the explanatory power of the resulting model. Yet, in those circumstances in which the survey is the obvious best option, reducing costs can often only be achieved by smaller or more focused samples, tighter questionnaires, using cheaper interview staff or limiting the depth of analysis. The various compromises have to be carefully weighed up against each other before embarking on the survey.

The two case examples offer illustrations of some of the dilemmas outlined above, and discuss the mistakes, limitations and longer term interpretation problems of surveys carried out within the time and resource constraints often present in policy and management oriented survey research.

CASE 1   HEALTH AND LIFESTYLE IN SOUTH SEFTON

The background

Britain has a long tradition of collating research material on the relationship between inequality and health (Illsley and Baker, 1991). It is matched by an equally long history of scholarly debate as to the causes of inequalities in health. The strongest proponent of the thesis that class and occupation are the primary determinants are Townsend and associates (Townsend and Davidson, 1982; Townsend *et al.*, 1988; Townsend, 1990; Townsend, 1991). Other researchers have supported his argument by examining widening social inequalities in the 1980s (Marmot and McDowall, 1986), assessing the decade after the publication of the Black report (Whitehead, 1987; Morris, 1990), reviewing research evidence on the nature and extent of social inequality in health and in outcomes of health care (Scott-Samuel, 1986), providing evidence that disadvantage in health status is related in a very regular way to the social class structure (Blaxter, 1987) or reviewing social inequalities within the context of a national health strategy (Delamothe, 1991).

Counter arguments have been formulated by Illsley and le Grand (1987) and Klein (1991) who argue that, indeed, serious inequalities exist but that occupational class is not necessarily the best analytical category on which to base theoretical explanations. They point out that 'over time the relative size of classes changes, i.e. that the significance and social meaning of inequalities change' (Klein, 1991, p.177). The domination of the class based argument has been questioned by researchers studying the relationship between structured disadvantage, gender and health status (Arber, 1991).

The continuing debate highlights not only the central importance of inequalities in health, but the complex issues involved in understanding causality. The fact that this debate is, as yet, unresolved is reflected in the publication of a national health strategy, carefully evading the issue altogether (DoH, 1991a and 1992) but being asked to account for that omission (Radical Statistics Group, 1991). Despite the disagreements about causal models, inequality is accepted as an important issue in understanding health and in formulating health policy.

It is within this climate that the national study on health and lifestyles was conceived. The introduction to the report states: 'When health is unequally distributed in society, as we know from the Black report, it is important to ask to what extent this is the result of differences in the experience of environments which induce vulnerability, or the relative failure of individuals in one part of the social spectrum to take adequate care of their health' (Cox *et al.*, 1987). It goes on to define the aims of the survey, attempting to assess the prevalence of particular patterns of health-related behaviour (diet, exercise, smoking and alcohol consumption) in various groups of the population and their associations with fitness and health. Furthermore, the beliefs which individuals hold about their health, and their attitudes to health and health promotion, are investigated, and the circumstances which may be relevant both to behaviour and to health – work, education, household structure, health history, and so on – are documented.

Blaxter (1990) specifies the strengths of this particular survey as offering the opportunity to look in a very general way at the relationship between attitudes, circumstances, behaviour and health. As such, it is a study of the general determinants of health, and a first attempt to consider the lives of individuals as a whole, with all the varied influences which bear upon their health (p.2).

The Health and Lifestyle Survey (HALS) was a national sample survey of men and women, of 18 years and over, living in private households in England, Wales and Scotland. The achieved sample size was 9003 people who were interviewed in 1984 and 1985. A second visit was made by a nurse who carried out a limited range of physiological measures, and who requested people to complete a further self-administered questionnaire, assessing personality and psychiatric status. The sampling frame used was the electoral register.

The South Sefton Health and Lifestyle Survey (SSHALS)

By the late 1980s community health services had moved towards a locally based assessment of the needs of their catchment populations. There was an increasing awareness that formulating a population's health profile on the basis of morbidity and mortality data was insufficient, as it focused on disease rather than health oriented thinking. In South Sefton, as in many other urban areas, health inequalities could be observed, and managers realized that understanding the differential experience of health would be an important aspect in health profiling.

In order to develop a programme of needs assessment capable of measuring the various dimensions of health, managers and researchers in South Sefton designed research consisting of qualitative and quantitative methodologies, each aimed at studying a different element of the health–disease complex. Thus, morbidity, mortality and deprivation indicators were analysed; GP populations studied, using validated tools such as the Nottingham Health Profile (Hunt *et al.*, 1986) and General Health Questionnaire (Goldberg and Hillier, 1979); the needs of specific client populations were conceptualized (discussed in Chapter Four); priorities were defined with local communities (discussed in Chapter Five) and normative needs were defined by professionals.

An important part of this total programme was a district-wide survey. Because South Sefton was divided into four localities which were distinct in their socio-economic composition, it was assumed that, as a result, the health needs in each locality would be different. At one end is the Bootle locality, where unemployment is high (30–36%), there is a low percentage of owner occupied housing (25–38%) and limited car ownership (22–35%); the other end of the spectrum is represented by Maghull locality with low rates of unemployment (7–13%), extensive home ownership (78–91%) and possession of a car (72–85%) (Klein, 1990).

For planning purposes a more detailed understanding of the socio-economic inequalities, and possibly related health inequalities, was needed to complement the above noted broad-based knowledge. Of particular interest were health promotion, stimulated by several successful local campaigns (for example, immunization and vaccination of the under-5s), and developments in primary care and mental health, because of the creation of community based facilities and preventive services. More generally, managers required an up-to-date baseline from which to formulate a strategic approach to community health.

The national HALS provided a suitable model for adaptation in the South Sefton context as it examined the relationship of lifestyles, behaviour and circumstances to the physical and mental health of populations. Thus, it met two objectives of South Sefton's managers: to provide a general picture of health, and to measure the most important components of the health experience, i.e. knowledge, attitudes, beliefs and behaviour within the context of socio-economic differences between the four localities. The SSHALS focused on specific areas of investigation which were topical for strategic planning. This meant that it took a more selective approach than the national HALS, also because of the considerably smaller available resources (Humphris *et al.*, 1990).

The SSHALS 'traded down' (Hakim, 1987) its design by reducing the number of issues to be investigated (that is, to focus on smoking, exercise and alcohol consumption), condense the questioning about specific disease patterns, include a limited number of questions about health beliefs, but add a few questions concerning people's caring status (in order to incorporate the concerns of Social Services colleagues). The wording of the questions remained unaltered in order to allow for maximum comparability with the national HALS.

The research was further traded down by using postgraduate students, following an applied research course at the university, as the inter- viewers and data processors, under the supervision of an experienced survey research lecturer. The costs of the survey included supervision, travel costs, production of the questionnaire, postage, computer time and printing 500 copies of the final report, and totalled £15 000 (1990 prices).

The sample

South Sefton has a population of 178 000 people (and declining). The survey population was defined as individuals on the electoral register, living in private households. Because the district was divided into four localities, and studying differences between these localities was a main objective, a stratified random sample was drawn from the four localities. From a total sample of 700 respondents the achieved sample size was 301, i.e. 43%. This very low response rate was due to the following factors:

1. In the areas of high mobility the electoral register is an unreliable basis for drawing a sample, because many people on the roll are no longer resident in the area. As a result, the Bootle and Netherton response rates were 37%.
2. In parts of the district security problems were very severe, and

people were reluctant to open the door. Furthermore, there was a general distrust of strangers, who could be tax collectors, bailiffs or other uninvited people, and this made gaining access more difficult for interviewers.

3. The survey was carried out in the winter months, when darkness falls around 5 pm. Older people (a high percentage living in the Crosby, Bootle and part of Maghull localities) and people living alone were reluctant to open the door after dark.

4. In Bootle several wards were under-represented in the original sample because of the inadequate electoral register information. Due to time constraints an alternative sampling strategy could not be developed, and extreme caution has to be applied when interpreting the results for this locality.

All respondents received an advance letter explaining the purpose of the interview, and indicating the period in which they would be visited. They were also given a contact address in case they wanted more information about the survey. Each address was visited three times (after which it was counted as a non-response). When a respondent agreed to be included in the study a structured interview was administered, lasting approximately 25 minutes.

The mainframe statistical package, SPSSX, was used to analyse the data. Statistical significance tests of probability have been carried out, and the standard interpretations used, i.e. $p < 0.05$ significant, $p < 0.01$ very significant. The main procedures used to test for significant associations and differences have been contingency table/Chi-square and ANOVA (analysis of variance). Whenever possible, similar subdivisions as in the national HALS have been used, but because of the smaller sample size, it has often been necessary to reduce the subcategories. The subdivision of particular interest in the SSHALS survey was the localities split, and data was analysed using this four-way distinction if at all possible.

Selected results

Blaxter (1990) discusses in detail the conceptual issues surrounding the notion of health, and the ways in which it is measured in the national HALS. She notes that health is a multidimensional concept incorporating professional and lay concepts of health. Understanding health directly relates to the theoretical and conceptual distinction between disease, which is defined as a biological abnormality, and illness, which is the subjective experience of the symptoms of ill health (Helman, 1990). The investigation into health needs has to take into account the 'objective' (clinical and medical diagnosis) and 'subjective' dimensions of health.

The HALS measured four dimensions of health, of which the SSHALS used three:

- disease and impairment or their absence, reflected in questions about limiting long-standing illness;
- experienced illness or freedom from illness, based on an index of symptoms suffered;
- psycho-social malaise or well-being, measured through symptoms which are predominantly psycho-social rather than physical (even though the distinction may be artificial) (Blaxter, 1990, pp.42–48) (Table 3.1).

The trend of increasing limiting disease with age is consistent with the national study, and the differences reported in the national HALS between social groupings are reflected in the differences between localities in the SSHALS (Table 3.2).

The two most affluent localities, Maghull and Crosby, report similar low levels of limiting disease, while the two other localities, Netherton and Bootle, report higher levels. However, the Bootle scores are substantially lower than Netherton whilst Bootle scores higher on the various deprivation indexes. Two explanations can be put forward: first, the Bootle population is younger (average 2 years younger than the Netherton sample); second, it is due to sampling error, which is the most likely reason.

The second method employed was to measure the presence of illness

Table 3.1 Degree of limiting disease (age, sex, locality)

		Age	
Males	18–39	40–59	60+
No disease	76	66	26
Non-limiting disease	13	5	24
Limiting disease	11	29	50
	100%	100%	100%
	(46)	(56)	(38)
Females			
No disease	84	68	52
Non-limiting disease	12	18	8
Limiting disease	4	14	40
	100%	100%	100%
	(56)	(50)	(50)

Table 3.2　Degree of limiting disease by locality

	Maghull	Crosby	Netherton/ Litherland	Bootle
No disease	73	69	53	57
Non-limiting disease	7	12	14	19
Limiting disease	20	19	33	24
	100%	100%	100%	100%
	(101)	(49)	(51)	(95)

Table 3.3　Prevalence reported during past month of selected symptoms

	Males Age			Females Age		
	18–39 %	40–59 %	60+ %	18–39 %	40–59 %	60+ %
Painful joints	15	39	45	10	34	44
Palpitations	13	12	39	14	12	28
Bad back	24	27	26	22	26	40
Trouble with feet	8	11	18	15	24	14
Trouble with eyes	13	18	31	15	14	30
Faints/dizziness	4	5	21	8	6	8
Constipation	6	7	10	19	12	16
Persistent cough	13	11	29	8	4	18
Sinus/catarrh	26	18	39	31	22	20
Indigestion	22	16	34	12	18	16
Headaches	52	22	34	51	48	34
Colds/flu	52	46	34	57	26	34
No. of respondents	46	56	38	58	50	50

through a checklist of common conditions which are particularly relevant in relation to lifestyle. The list of symptoms are the most frequent as reported in extensive general practitioner surveys. While it is recognized that checklists can result in over-reporting, and that bias can arise out of not interviewing people with more serious disease because they are not cared for at home, these self-defined disease categories can be helpful in understanding what people consider to be health problems (Table 3.3).

The overall trends are similar to the national HALS in that with increasing age more symptoms are reported, with the exception of headaches, colds and flu. But on the whole, the South Sefton population reports more symptoms than the national sample: for example, painful joints are almost twice as likely to occur in the two lower age bands, and men in South Sefton appear to suffer from back trouble right through life at the level of the oldest age band in the national survey. When analysed alongside the other evidence about prescribed drugs, people in South Sefton seem to feel less healthy than in the national study, which in all probability will be borne out in the demand for health and social services.

The SSHALS focused on the concept of malaise by using a composite score of self-perceived psycho-social symptoms: difficulty sleeping, always feeling tired, difficulty concentrating, worrying 'over every little thing', 'nerves', feeling bored, feeling 'under so much strain that your health is likely to suffer'. The last three categories received extra weight when answered 'always'. The categories used in the table are:

- high malaise: 4+ symptoms;
- average malaise: 2/3 symptoms;
- low malaise: 0/1 symptom (Table 3.4).

The biggest difference with the national HALS is that the younger age group reports higher levels of malaise. For males the difference is 23% in the national sample against 33% in South Sefton; for females, 34%

Table 3.4 Incidence of specific symptoms of 'malaise' during last month (age/ sex)

	Males Age			Females Age		
	18–39 %	40–59 %	60+ %	18–39 %	40–59 %	60+ %
Difficulty sleeping	28.2	21.4	31.6	39.6	30.0	30.0
Always feel tired	28.2	19.6	15.7	37.9	30.0	20.0
Worrying over every little thing	15.2	12.5	18.4	32.7	32.0	28.0
Nerves	8.7	8.9	10.5	18.9	26.0	24.0
Difficulty concentrating	28.3	8.9	13.2	17.2	22.0	12.0
Bored	4.3	12.5	13.3	20.6	8.0	10.0
Lonely	2.2	5.3	15.8	10.3	4.0	16.0
Under strain	4.3	8.9	5.3	13.8	18.0	6.0
No. of respondents	46	56	38	58	50	50

against 43%. When analysing the detail, the younger men in South Sefton report higher levels of difficulty sleeping and always feeling tired. Females in South Sefton present with a reverse picture than the national sample: in South Sefton, younger women report more difficulty sleeping than older women, and similarly score higher on worry and being under strain. It appears that there is a generally higher level of malaise, in particular among the younger age group, than would be expected from the national picture. This is consistent with the priorities defined by local communities in Bootle who see mental health promotion as an important area of work (see Chapter Five).

The national HALS reported a link between unemployment and malaise, which has also been documented elsewhere (Smith, 1987). The SSHALS confirms this picture, with high malaise amongst those not working part- or full-time (Table 3.5).

Perceptions of health were a central element in the national HALS, and partially studied in the SSHALS. Here, one aspect is discussed, namely what people felt affected their health and whether they were actively involved in taking control over their own health. This latter question was divided into what people considered to be activities which one would ideally like to engage in, and what people actually managed to put into health promoting practice. Thus, the analysis focused on understanding the discrepancy, if any, between intended and actual behaviour. This issue is important when considering the impact of information and education, and the existence of opportunities to behave in ways that are consistent with knowledge. It was hypothesized that people's so-called unhealthy behaviour was not the result of ignorance, but rather the lack of opportunities in a financial sense, availability of services, low self-image and so on (Jacobson *et al.*, 1991).

Two types of questions were asked: first, 'Do you do anything at the moment to keep yourself healthy or improve your health?'; second, 'Are there any things you would like to do to keep yourself healthy but don't

Table 3.5 Malaise and employment

	Not working part or full-time	Working part or full-time
Low malaise	28	36
Average malaise	32	37
High malaise	40	27
	100%	100%
	(151)	(146)

do?' followed by 'if "yes" what would you like to do?'. In the SSHALS a simple cumulative score was calculated for both questions; the results are shown in Figure 3.1.

Comparing intentions – which is a proxy of knowledge about health enhancing activities – the people in Netherton and Maghull displayed similar levels, whilst the people in Crosby scored higher. When comparing the actual activities Maghull's respondents did considerably more than the Netherton respondents. The differences in socio-economic status, and therefore the relative lack of financial resources available for health promoting activities such as sport and exercise, could be a contributive factor for Netherton's lower score. Furthermore, facilities in Netherton are considered to be sparse, certainly when compared to Crosby and Maghull. For managers, the priority was not to put more resources into educating the general public, but to investigate further the reasons why people were not able to pursue health activities and to devise alternative ways in which to offer health services.

The SSHALS was a modest exercise, and some of the main problems with the execution of the survey have been discussed. Despite its limitations and shortcomings, the survey proved to be a useful complement to the other research tools aimed at building up a picture of health and health care needs. It certainly helped managers to focus on key areas of change or service development. Furthermore, it provided a baseline for regular (re-)assessment of needs, and to assist in the possible formulation of outcomes of population-based interventions.

There are, of course, many other research tools that could have been applied, but an important argument has been to use tools that have proven to be scientifically robust. The national HALS served as an important comparative base for the local analysis of data, and a survey designed specifically for South Sefton would not benefit from such a comparison. In general, managers do not have the time or resources to develop research tools from scratch, and would be well advised to use reliable and validated instruments which save time and are more likely to yield strong material.

CASE 2   DEVELOPING A USER FEEDBACK SURVEY

Having argued that validated instruments are the most cost-effective choice, there are, of course, situations in which current knowledge is rudimentary, and it is necessary to develop new research approaches. One such area is user feedback research.

The structural changes in health services in western Europe and North America have stimulated the debate about the question of whether users should be consulted about aspects of service delivery. McIver (1991) argues that there is probably an acceptance among service purchasers

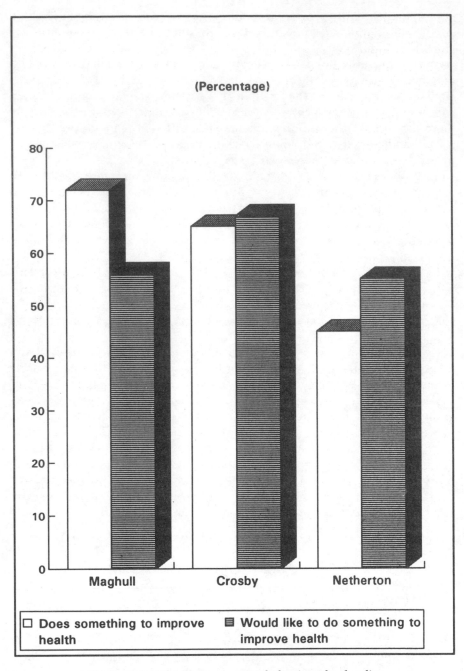

(Percentage)

☐ Does something to improve health   ▤ Would like to do something to improve health

Figure 3.1 Health improving behaviour by locality

and providers that users' views are necessary for evaluating and improving quality. At the same time, the process of obtaining those views is complicated and riddled with controversy (Stimson and Webb, 1975; Fitzpatrick and Hopkins, 1983). This is partly because the field is relatively new for the health care context, and only a few systematic studies have been undertaken (Raphael, 1977; Cartwright and Anderson, 1982; Thompson, 1983) which produced tools that are more generally applicable. Moreover, the majority of studies have employed a narrow focus, examining the notion of patient satisfaction, without necessarily defining the concept itself (Locker and Dunt, 1979).

Indirectly, the issue of satisfaction has been addressed by Thompson (1983) who found some evidence to support the classic theory of satisfaction which was largely based on non-health settings. He argues that the sources of satisfaction are qualitatively different from the sources of dissatisfaction; that is, the absence of satisfaction with an aspect of a service does not directly imply the existence of dissatisfaction, or vice versa. If applied to health settings, managers should not uncritically respond to survey findings which emphasize negative aspects of the service, because dissatisfaction would not directly be influenced. Rather, a concentration on the positive aspects of care could effect a considerable increase in satisfaction.

McIver (1991) points out a further issue which warrants attention, namely the distinction between asking users to evaluate the process of service delivery and asking about outcome. Furthermore, she argues that asking people about what they feel they need is again a separate question. Taken together, these considerations demonstrate the conceptual difficulties surrounding the notion of satisfaction.

It is important to understand that the key problem is subjectivity, namely, the subjective assessment of service quality on the part of the user. This subjectivity has to be understood before we can make any statements about satisfaction or dissatisfaction, as they constitute only a part of the totality of user perceptions.

Surveying satisfaction in two regional specialties

In 1991 West Midlands Regional Health Authority (WMRHA) commissioned the Centre for Health Planning and Management to develop a user satisfaction tool for use in regional specialties. The first two specialties to be piloted were radiotherapy and renal services.

The research was a multistaged study consisting of:

1. literature review on general and specific instruments of satisfaction/feedback;

2. a series of ethnographic interviews with key actors in order to formulate the main areas of user feedback;
3. observation of clinics;
4. the design of a structured questionnaire to be administered to samples of patients in order to test construct validity and internal reliability;
5. repeat administration of structured questionnaire to a smaller subsample from 4 above in order to measure test/retest reliability.

A literature review is a conventional preliminary stage almost invariably applied in research projects, and which is intended to place the current research in the context of past work in related fields. The research literature concerning the experience of illness has covered various cancers (Higginson *et al.*, 1990; Pritchard, 1988) and renal disease (Gerhardt, 1990). However, studies on user feedback within the two specialties were sparse and, as a result, the WMRHA project decided to design and test a tailor-made instrument.

The observations and ethnographic interviews were the first stage in this development process. Interviews were carried out with a selected number of consultants in the region. It was attempted to achieve representative coverage, relying on the advice of the specialists in the Research Steering Group (set up specifically for this project), which resulted in five consultant radiotherapists and oncologists, and three renal specialists being interviewed. Furthermore, registrars, haemodialysis and CAPD (continuous ambulatory peritoneal dialysis) nurses, radiographers and radiotherapy/oncology nurses were interviewed. The format followed was a loosely structured discussion ranging from factual description of the type and level of service provision to a conceptual understanding of the patient's experience of illness and the response required from clinicians. Organizational issues such as access and multidisciplinary working were addressed. Coverage of these areas was aimed at describing what service providers thought were important indicators of patient satisfaction.

The selection of patients was more complex because their experiences of illness and service provision depended on the stage of their disease, and the attendant treatments. The literature also pointed to the significance of social and economic variables. Thus, a matrix of key characteristics was drawn up for each patient population, which in the case of cancer patients contained the following dimensions:

- type of therapy: radiotherapy or chemotherapy;
- the absence or presence of informal support;
- the type of cancer: at this stage only breast cancer and lung cancer patients were included.

Eight selected patients, each representing a cell in the matrix, drawn from two appropriate pilot sites, were interviewed using the ethnographic interview schedule.

The renal patients sample was derived in a similar way, drawing on the following dimensions:

- employment career: unemployed/retired or employe ! outside the home;
- treatment career: hospital or home dialysis, CAPD;
- the absence or presence of informal support.

Twelve patients were interviewed in two pilot sites.

All 20 respondents were approached by their own specialist and asked for their consent to be interviewed by the researchers. The interviews took place in people's own homes, and were tape-recorded and transcribed. The qualitative analysis was aimed to generate a number of issues or indicators which could be translated into items for a structured questionnaire.

The results are schematically represented in Figures 3.2 and 3.3.

Conventional outpatients satisfaction surveys concentrate on issues surrounding waiting times and physical surroundings. The regional specialties study revealed this to be just one component of a larger complex. The four main areas of concern are represented in Figures 3.2 and 3.3, but not all these areas were similarly emphasized. For example, consultants and users placed stress upon the content and timing of information, whilst radiographers and nurses focused on the organization of care.

There were important differences between the two diseases. For example, information for cancer patients centred around knowledge about the nature and stage of the disease, different treatment regimens and especially the explanation of side effects. Renal patients felt that the timing of information was important in order that they could assess the impact of dialysis on their lifestyle. The complexity of the patient 'career' (Goffman, 1961) was confirmed through the ethnographic analysis: cancer patients could have had surgery or not, received radiotherapy or chemotherapy or both, and these various treatments could have different chronological patterns. Similarly, renal patients could have experienced CAPD, home or hospital dialysis in different sequences, sometimes interspersed with a failed kidney transplant. The study assumed that a user's satisfaction with a particular mode of treatment might be influenced by prior experience of this or other modes.

Given these considerations, the development of a structured user feedback instrument had to be sufficiently complex in order to incorporate the dimensions and layers of the experience of illness,

Surveys in health services research

Groups of Interviewees

	Consultants	Radiographers	Nursing Staff	Chemotherapy Patients	Radiotherapy Patients
INFORMATION TO PATIENTS	Accurate, truthful, immediate	Reiteration. Elaboration of earlier info.	Elaboration.	Side-effects. Written info.	Information specialist role. Info on range of treatments.
ORGANISATION OF CARE	Speed of total process.	Waiting time. Physical environment. Transport. Continuity.	Waiting time. Physical environment. Continuity of care.	Time given. Privacy. Choice. Staff turn-over.	Time given. Waiting time. Physical environment.
ASSESSMENT OF PERSONNEL	Caring staff. Accessibility. Professionalism	Friendly caring staff.	Positive staff attitudes.	Consultant style. Staff attitudes.	Style. Accessibility.
SUPPORT FOR PATIENT AND/ OR FAMILY	Supportive staff. Home support.	Counselling. Home support. Non-medical support.	Counselling. Nurse back-up. Phone line.	Counselling. Support groups. Social work.	Support groups. Counselling.

From: Ong and Shiels, 1991

Figure 3.2 Radiotherapy/oncology: main satisfaction issues stressed by groups of interviewees

Groups of Interviewees

	Consultants	Haemodialysis Nurses	CAPD Nurses	CAPD Patients	Haemodialysis Patients
INFORMATION TO PATIENT.	Early prognosis. Limitations to choice.	Reiteration of info. Written info.	Info on all aspects of CAPD.	Pre-dialysis info. Limitations of CAPD. Simple booklet.	Impact on lifestyle. Access to all relevant info.
ORGANISATION OF CARE.	Flexibility of treatment. Style of delivery.	Full assessment of patient. Flexibility. Waiting times.	Full training. Flexibility. Continuity of care.	Choice of treatment. Time given to patient. Waiting times.	Back-up treatment. Flexibility. Waiting. Transport.
ASSESSMENT OF PERSONNEL.	Positive staff attitudes.	Stability of patient-nurse relationship. Accessibility of senior staff.	Rapport between patient and community staff.	Caring clinic staff.	Atmosphere on unit. Individual attention.
SUPPORT FOR PATIENT AND/ OR FAMILY.	Home support. Family support. Counselling/ psychiatric input.	Counselling. Support groups. Family needs.	Practical and emotional support for patient and family.	Home visits. Telephone contact. Counselling. Support groups.	Counselling. Social worker. Support groups.

From: Ong and Shiels, 1991

Figure 3.3 Renal dialysis: main satisfaction issues stressed by groups of interviewees

treatment processes and outcomes. Yet, at the same time, it had to be in a format suitable for self-completion of large samples, and easy to analyse for health service managers.

The structured questionnaire

Two questionnaires have been constructed using a modular approach. In the case of renal services, the questionnaire starts with a section on their dialysis to be filled in by all patients; the second module asks about general satisfaction with the treatment process followed by optional modules covering GAPD and hospital haemodialysis, with a concluding module for all patients asking a few personal details. The radiotherapy questionnaire has a similar format with optional modules for radiotherapy and chemotherapy.

WMRHA commissioned a structured instrument which can be used as a management tool, which led the researchers to devise some form of satisfaction index (or indices) compiled from aggregating item scores in the questionnaire. Such an index could lead to useful comparisons across sites and specialties, and at one site or within a specialty over time (Shiels, 1991).

In order to establish the questionnaire as a tested and sensitive instrument, capable of being used over time and across different sites and/or specialties, three tests had to be conducted:

1. Construct validity: this test attempts to establish whether the instrument is really measuring what it aims to do; that is, whether it can demonstrate variations in satisfaction levels across different sites. Therefore, two sites which vary in terms of organization of care, staff levels, support services, appointment systems, etc. were chosen for each specialty and the questionnaires were to be administered to subsamples in those locations. The questionnaire should pick up variations in satisfaction levels, and the statistical tests used for ascertaining these included the T-test, Kruskal–Wallis test, analysis of variance and the Mann–Whitney U-test.
2. Internal reliability: as items in the questionnaire are to be combined into an overall index it has to be tested whether all the items are indeed valid indicators of the total concept of satisfaction. Thus, respondents' answers should show consistency across questions of a similar nature in the various modules, and the statistical test used is the Cronbach's alpha test.
3. Test/retest reliability: the questionnaire should have the ability to be used on the same subject group over time, which means that a test of the instrument's external reliability has to be carried out. The subsamples received the questionnaire at two points in time, with a

sufficiently long intervening period. Providing that, in the meantime, there have been no changes in the delivery of care that might affect satisfaction, there should be a strong correlation between index scores and individual satisfaction ratings measured at different points in time. The statistical tests used are Pearson's correlation test and Spearman's rank coefficient (see Shiels, 1991 and 1992a for more details).

The latter stages of the project require statistical expertise and access to SPSS (PC or mainframe) facilities. However, the production of a reliable and validated tool which takes time and resources means that it can be used as a continuous user-feedback instrument, and extended to other regional specialties.

The WMRHA user feedback project has produced a validated survey tool that can be used as a management tool in the region, and as such has generalized and longer term value for planning purposes. The tool has been supported by a series of documents covering methodological issues, a user manual (SPSS) and a step-by-step guide for managers implementing the survey in their service. It has been acknowledged by regional managers that such a survey requires their direct involvement in the implementation stage so as to clearly define its strategic significance. These types of tools cannot just be implemented from above but have to be linked with management concerns such as monitoring performance and contract specifications.

CONCLUSION

Surveys can be applied across a range of problems, and are capable of studying large groups of people. As such, they are very attractive for health managers. But because surveys amass a relatively large quantity of data they tend to be costly in time and resources. Strategic planning requires both short and long time horizons, and it is important to ascertain the utility of surveys within those two different time frames. Furthermore, because surveys are expensive, other cheaper methods or 'traded down' designs should be carefully considered before opting for a survey.

Surveys tend to produce information that is less detailed, but can be applied fairly confidently over a broad area (Giddens, 1989). Thus, the first case example provided an overall picture of the health of a district, without being able to assign causality or give complex explanations of the relationships between beliefs, attitudes, social circumstances and geographical location. Yet, the broad brush approach allowed the emergence of a series of issues which required closer examination and which were able to focus management thinking; for example, questioning the emphasis of health promotion on education instead of on facilitating the participation in health promoting activities.

The second example illustrated the application of surveys in user feedback research and discussed the way in which an instrument had to be tested for validity and reliability before being confidently administered across large and varied patient populations. In general, managers and researchers are well advised to use tools that are already validated and for which comparative findings exist. However, in new fields such as user feedback this is not always possible and suitable instruments have to be devised. The case example showed that the development of a measure is a laborious process, requiring considerable statistical expertise. Managers have to decide whether the investment is cost-effective, which was the case with the regional specialties research because the instrument was not exclusively intended for the two pilot specialties.

Many people in the health service use the term surveys in a loose and often inaccurate manner, and as a result tend to underestimate the complexity of carrying out sound research. At the same time, the survey method is one of the most extensively documented methodologies, and some of the literature has been referred to in this chapter. For the health context the Cartwright and Seale volume (1990) is extremely useful because it highlights all the key stages of the survey, and managers and researchers would be wise to consult this book before embarking on a survey themselves.

Chapter Four

Ethnography in health services research

INTRODUCTION

Qualitative research, and in particular ethnography, has traditionally been considered as representing anthropology *par excellence*. The perception that the ethnographer has to 'go native', immersing him or herself in the local culture, dominated lay understanding, and as a result managers saw it as an esoteric and uneconomical way of studying the organizational problems they were faced with. The knowledge generated by ethnography was considered to be idiographic, which implied that there was a problem of confidence in the generalizability of findings. The emergence of specific case studies in health policy and management which draw on ethnographic principles has demonstrated the value of this approach in understanding subjectivity, experiences and processes, all important aspects of human relations in organizations.

This chapter discusses the principles and use of ethnography in health research by way of two case studies. The first case study concerns a key area in health service management, namely organizational change. It is now commonplace to say that the health service is undergoing constant change but, as yet, understanding of change processes is incomplete (Strong and Robinson, 1990) and managers do not systematically apply scientific methodologies for investigating what happens within their organizations. As a result, important lessons are lost and managers are 'reinventing the wheel' time and time again.

Turning to established social science methodologies for the examination of processes of change helps to identify similarities and differences of various reorganizations in order to build up insights which can guide subsequent processes. Furthermore, developing outcome measures of successful organizational change is an important area of enquiry for strategic management. We will discuss the nature, methods and possible outcomes of ethnography in the study of organizations, arguing that this qualitative approach is capable of uncovering the complexity and richness necessary for grasping the totality of the process of change at organizational and individual levels, and the interaction between the two.

The second case study focuses on assessing users' needs for particular services. In Bradshaw's taxonomy of need (1972) the distinction between the professional and managerial definitions, based on normative and comparative notions, and user led definitions, based on felt and expressed needs, offers a conceptual framework. Studying users' and carers' own experience of health and illness provides the opportunity to compare their assessment of needs with those grounded in professional standard setting and resource management.

The Griffiths Inquiry of 1983 marked the beginning of a new relationship between the general managers and the professions, and has been documented in various pieces of research (Strong and Robinson, 1990; Small, 1989; Paton and Bach, 1990). The tensions between the aims of the service, decision-making processes and professional autonomy are the obvious areas of research. Yet, the role of research in facilitating this major attitudinal and organizational shift has been relatively neglected.

Research on organizational decision-making has questioned the established paradigm that there is a linear progression from decision-making to action. Instead, it is argued that there is often a gap between statements of intent and operational implementation, and that decision-making needs to be seen as a continuous process (Pettigrew, 1990). In the context of the health service, with different power groups existing alongside each other, this is particularly relevant. Conflict of interest, opposing philosophies and strategies, and different frameworks of interpretation all interface in the continuum between statements of intent and implementation.

When health services embark on a process of organizational change, in-depth understanding of the social systems of managers, professionals and other staff groups is essential. The differentiation of functions, how roles and responsibilities are created, re-created and maintained, identifying the dominant values and emerging expectations are all elements which require to be understood if targeting, implementing and consolidating change are to be successful.

Designing research capable of supporting organizational change has to be aimed at understanding the internal dynamics of the organization. An important element within that is conceptualizing the unfolding perceptions in key actors as the main movers behind change processes and acceptance of change (Isabella, 1990). Ethnographic methods are suited to this aim as they tend to focus on a single case or a small number of cases to be studied in depth and within context (Yin, 1984) in order to capture 'still frames' of an organization at different moments in time. A 'moving picture' can be built up through the collection of a wide variety of data about many properties which help to gain detailed comprehension of the system under scrutiny.

Hammersley and Atkinson (1983) describe the ethnographic researcher as someone who 'participates, overtly or covertly, in people's daily lives for an extended period of time, watching what happens, listening to what is said, asking questions; in fact collecting whatever data are available to throw light on the issues with which he or she is concerned' (p.2). Applying this to the health service manager, Strong and Robinson (1990) argue that, in order to understand their own organization, managers engage in ethnography because 'he or she walks the patch, chats with other staff, goes to meetings, scrutinises documents, watches how others behave, swaps notes with friends and other observers. . .' (p.7). Yet, this knowledge is not always made explicit or used systematically. Only when the collection of data proceeds as a planned exercise, using techniques such as 'snowballing' or comparing and contrasting various data sets so that evidence is accumulated which allows a multifaceted examination of the problem in hand, can this be called research.

Managers can employ different strategies for using ethnographic research in the planning, implementation and monitoring of organizational change. Outsiders can research the organization (Strong and Robinson, 1990; Alaszewski and Ong, 1990; Pettigrew *et al.*, 1992); managers themselves do formal or informal research (Roberts, 1992) or researchers are integrated within the management structure to do 'research from within' (Ong, 1989). It is the latter approach that is discussed in the case study.

One of the cornerstones of ethnography is observation, participant or non-participant (Spradley, 1980; Whyte, 1984), which is a specific method characterized by the 'immersion of the researcher into the system under analysis'. Participant observation employs observation, informal questioning and recording 'hearsay'. Thus, a dynamic research model combining different and flexible data collection strategies is developed capable of studying the processes of change and adaptation taking place and understanding the internal system and relationships within and with outsiders.

Non-participant observation makes the above processes more explicit and the researcher is known to operate within the system as a researcher. It has been argued that this mode of operation creates the 'Hawthorne effect' whereby, through intruding on the research situation itself, or by heightening the participant's awareness that they are under study, one runs the risk of changing the very action that is under observation (Riley, 1963, p.628). Contrary to this argument it can be said that in lengthy periods of observation participants cannot continue to 'act', and the Hawthorne effect will diminish.

Giddens (1989) argues that social sciences are scientific disciplines, in the sense that they involve systematic methods of investigation, the analysis of data and the assessment of theories in the light of evidence and logical argument. At the same time, one has to realize that social scientists study human beings and social life, which is meaningful to the people engaged in social activities. A key characteristic of ethnography is that it does not attempt to modify behaviour but, by 'getting under people's skin', tries to examine 'meaningful behaviour'. Using this approach of 'Verstehen' (emphatic understanding) organizational change can be designed in a more scientific manner. Combining the study of meaning with assessing the impact of policy initiatives throws light on how new ideas are built on existing frames of reference, identifies key actors and agents of change and locates the nature and sources of resistance. The scientific basis for policy change can be strengthened through analysing different models of practice and strategies for change. The two case studies illustrate this ethnographic policy application.

CASE 1   CHANGING MENTAL HEALTH SERVICES

The background

Changes in mental health services since the introduction of general management are particularly interesting as they coincide with major conceptual shifts in the aims and objectives of the services generally, resulting in professional and government-led re-orientations. This combination of theoretical and policy shifts instigated complex processes of adaptation in individuals and organizations. The study of the contextual experience of change using ethnographic methods could assist in the formulation of strategies aimed at redirecting mental health services.

The paradigmatic changes in mental health have been largely the result of academic initiated work on institutions (Goffman, 1961); of subsequent theoretical developments in related fields such as the normalization philosophy adapted from mental handicap services (Wolfensberger, 1983; O'Brien and Tyne, 1981) and as a reaction to international experiments such as the radical moves to community based psychiatry in Italy (Ramon, 1987). As a result, the medical model has come under scrutiny and the social aspects of mental health are increasingly being emphasized, with some adopting a medically based model (Kuipers, 1987), others departing into a social constructivist model (Ingleby, 1983).

The relationship between inequality and mental health has been forcefully argued by authors focusing on specific social groups such as ethnic minorities (Torkington, 1991) or researchers studying the treatment of women (Busfield, 1989). This body of work created pressure on the theoretical underpinnings of the medical model which drew parallels with the general theory of disturbance in the body's normal functioning, and instead focused on social, cultural and economic disturbance. The dominance of the psychiatrists in the provision of mental health was questioned and the skills provided by nurses, social workers, psychologists, occupational therapists, welfare rights workers and voluntary organizations had to be recognized.

Psychiatrists argue that because of the introduction of major tranquillizers and the subsequent successful control of many disturbances a shift to the social origins of mental illness has been possible. They consider the medical foundation as the cornerstone of care, and view the input of other approaches as complementary, but subordinate to the medico-psychiatric model.

Alongside the above changes public concerns about the care of people with mental health problems emerged in the late 1960s as a result of a series of scandals about the provision of care. Since then, subsequent governments have embarked on a programme of running down large mental health institutions (DHSS,1962; DHSS, 1975) while aiming to expand community-based services. However, the success of building up alternative services was severely criticized in the Audit Commission's report (1986).

The report demonstrated that there had been slow movement towards the targets set by the 1975 White Paper, and that the build-up of community-based services was running behind the reduction of hospital provisions. The Commission highlighted many other organizational problems such as gross geographical variations, perverse economic incentives and complex structures and multiple agency providers.

The Audit Commission report was a precursor to the subsequent Griffiths report (1988) and the *White Paper Caring for People* (DoH, 1989a). The latter two documents were inspired by new service developments, most notably the care manager model, which is based on the assessment of the needs of individual clients in order to design a flexible and individually tailored 'package of care' (Beardshaw and Towell, 1990; Allen, 1990).

The result of this government-led pressure was the move to decentralized services for people with mental health problems, and a multidisciplinary, multi-agency approach to care. Furthermore, serious attention had to be given to involving users and their social networks in the planning and evaluation of services.

The combination of theoretical and organizational change in mental health services created a complex process of adaptation, at both an individual and an organizational level. Understanding how people and social systems coped with these pressures and how best change could be planned needed a clear strategy, underpinned by research into the workings of the service.

South Sefton Mental Health: a case example

In 1987, as a result of the introduction of general management South Sefton Health Authority (SSHA) formed a new unit combining priority (mental health, mental handicap and elderly services) with community services. At that point, the Mental Health Unit continued to operate with a professional-based management system: Director of Nursing Services, Nursing Officers and Sisters and Charge Nurses, alongside the separate Psychiatric Division which 'organized' the psychiatrists. Occupational Therapy and Psychology were managed by District Heads, accountable to the UGM, and social work was managed through the Local Authority.

The Unit, like many others nationally, was subject to the shifts discussed previously: changing ideas about the causes of mental health problems created tensions between the various professional groups and their respective contributions; centrally directed changes in patterns of service provisions gave rise to uncertainties and moving alliances.

Locally, three catalysts for change could be identified: firstly, the run down of the large mental institution which traditionally cared for the catchment population by detaining people with long-term needs. As a receiving District, plans for the replacement of a range of services had to be drawn up and put into operation ready for the planned hospital closure by 1991. Secondly, the Unit had been given the task of designing a new 125-bed acute hospital to be built on the DGH site by September 1988, and transferring all acute services to be housed in the new unit. Thirdly, a new Director of Nursing Services was appointed in April 1987 to oversee the two major changes, and with the additional task of implementing general management within the Mental Health Unit.

The Unit, consistent with the national picture, suffered from problems directly related to financial stringency on the one hand, and an authoritarian structure on the other. As a result many staff were demoralized and left. Staff development was absent, and new ideas were not encouraged to come up from the grass roots. In short, the hallmarks of a backward organization were in evidence.

After the creation of the new unit the Unit General Manager (UGM) and Director of Nursing Services (DNS) started by drawing up a philosophy of care for mental health services, appointed a Manager of Human Resources (MHR) in charge of staff training and development and a Manager of Research and Development (MRD), both recruited to support the process of change.

The newly formulated philosophy of care reflected the progressive ideas about mental health services, emphasizing the principles of normalization, defining care as a holistic and continuous process, creating better communication and integration with other services and individuals. Putting the philosophy of care into operation needed the decentralization of management to ward level in order to bring decision-making closer to the client. Central to the development of new ideas and their subsequent implementation was the team approach to the management of change. The process of change was a multidisciplinary endeavour, and explicitly defined the research element as an agent of change.

Ethnography as a diagnostic tool

In a recent debate on the nature and methods of ethnography Hammersley (1990) argues that ethnographic descriptions depend on what we believe to be true and on judgements about relevance, which are directly related to the purposes which the description is to serve. He goes on to argue that the relevances and the factual and value assumptions that underlie any specific ethnographic descriptions and explanations have to be made explicit. This reasoning is important when employing ethnography within a management context, where the objectives for research are jointly defined with managers in order to achieve system change.

In the South Sefton case the impetus for changing services was generated by the introduction of general management, but reinforced by the need to rethink the paradigms current in mental health practice. At the same time, resistance against change was strongly motivated from within the psychiatric and nursing professions, because of the threat to professional control and attendant professional status which needed to be protected. As a result, the aims of research as an agent of change had to be carefully formulated, and clearly distinguished from organizational development consultancy work. The scientific approach was emphasized by carrying out a separate investigation of theories on the nature and treatment of mental health problems, an assessment of current structures of control, and subjective experiences of the service. This was opera-tionalized into the following components:

- Research into good models of practice could provide a scientific argument for alternative ways of providing services, which were able to demonstrate quality and successful outcomes.
- An analysis of the present organization, its management structures, its operation and service delivery was intended to illustrate the strengths and weaknesses of current practices, and point to oppor-tunities for change.

- The examination of attitudes and perceptions was seen as an important element of organizational diagnosis in defining paradigmatic shifts which could set the agenda for addressing key service themes.

Thus, the agenda was explicitly defined by managers who wanted to realign the service in keeping with general management principles. The researcher's role was to build the scientific basis for this change, shape it according to good practice at the 'leading edge', and provide guidance for the change process as a whole. The research design, therefore, contained an analysis of secondary data sources, outlining principles and practices of new and innovative developments in mental health. From this literature research certain projects could be earmarked for more intensive investigation, by either collecting documentary evidence or by examining them directly through observation and interviewing.

The organizational diagnosis was structured to combine observation of different service settings with formal and informal questioning of participants, including users and carers. Following the two main research strategies, observation and questioning, steering and monitoring the change process was the next phase.

Observation

The distinction between participant and non-participant observation cannot easily be drawn when doing research within a organizational change framework (Ong, 1989). In the role of researcher networks of actions and reactions among group members can be studied, which will uncover patterns of interaction and role structures. However, there is also a degree of participation in reflecting on the organization and formulating emerging ideas about change which requires a closer relationship with group members, and being drawn into their worlds. Clear delineation between a research activity, such as studying ward records, and more participatory activities, such as taking part in occupational therapy group sessions, has to be made in order to allow both types of data collection to take place.

The research started in September 1987 with studying models of care in rehabilitation. Simultaneously, the first stage of observations was initiated, comprising a series of visits to all wards and departments covering periods which were representative of the type of work carried out. Therefore, visits to acute wards were carried out during the day when occupational therapy sessions took place, as well as during the evening and night. Group work in the day hospitals was observed and clinics in outpatient departments. Ward rounds and meetings were attended, and client meetings on the acute wards. The researcher accompanied CPNs on domiciliary visits. A couple of meetings of the relatives support group were attended.

Hammersley (1992) offers a critique of ethnography as 'insightful' description, presuming there exists a single, objective description of a particular phenomenon. Instead, he states that multiple and contradictory truths exist, and for ethnography to be relevant its purpose has to be made explicit. In this case ethnographic observations served to uncover structures between the medical and nursing professionals and within each discipline. Consistent with other studies about medical and nursing hierarchies (Freidson,1975; Strong, 1979; Stacey, 1988) the mental health environment showed similar patterns. The organization of the ward was geared towards the working methods of the psychiatrists, with the ward rounds as the organizing principle. The interactions in the ward round were orchestrated by the psychiatrist, who interrogated the client and invited observations from nursing staff as and when deemed necessary.

The shifting conceptions of the causes of mental ill health incorporating the socio-psychological elements could potentially have undermined the medical model in psychiatry, and with it the dominant structural position of the psychiatrist. The observations demonstrated the opposite: the medical model was strongly invoked in diagnosing causality and determining treatment. The use of drugs outweighed the referral to psychologists, whilst social work, occupational therapy and nursing were perceived as supplementing medical interventions.

The organization of nursing mirrored the medical hierarchy and strict boundaries between 'trained' and 'untrained' and day and night staff were maintained. This meant a loss of knowledge, and stifling initiative and development of skills. Communications between the various staff groups were often deficient, resulting in lack of co-ordination and inconsistencies in care. Staff lower down the hierarchy were rarely asked for their opinion, often were not informed of decisions and generally felt devalued. Care planning was done by trained staff with little or no systematic involvement of untrained nurses or other professionals.

Paralleling the lack of involvement of junior members of staff in decision-making processes was the symbolic participation of clients. Client meetings tended to focus on procedural matters, but did not incorporate notions of self-advocacy and critical assessment of the services provided (Patmore, 1989). As in most health service organizations, involving the users did not go beyond a 'patient satisfaction' approach by asking people to make choices about issues that were peripheral to the policies and operation of the unit.

The authoritarian and medically dominated system resulted in a feeling among the majority of staff that their ideas were not valued, that there was no commitment to developing people and that management seemed to accept low staffing levels, which led to delivering minimal care. Innovation and creativity, especially involving grassroots staff and clients, were not encouraged. The organization as a whole suffered from low morale, staff turnover was great and patterns of working reinforced existing hierarchies and conservative ideas.

Observation allowed the collection of data which reflected the network of actions and reactions amongst the people observed. At the same time the process of observation itself was seen by the various staff groups as an important vehicle for conveying their experiences to managers. In their eyes the research could be used to demonstrate the way in which the service operated, and the role of the different professional groups within it. Staff continually stressed that this first hand knowledge ratified their aspirations, or in their own words, 'now you have seen it for yourself'. This placed the researcher in the position of a mediator between staff and managers. Credibility had to be maintained both with staff and managers for the research to make an impact on policy formulation. It was, therefore, crucially important to maintain a certain scientific independence, in order not to be drawn into specific power struggles.

Questioning

Questioning has been a fundamental method within social science research, and all classic methodology textbooks deal with the various techniques. Oakley, in her insightful critique of interviewing, summarizes the dominant paradigm of the social research interview as one that emphasizes:

- its status as a mechanical instrument of data collection;
- its function as a specialized form of conversation in which one person asks the questions and another gives the answers;
- its characterization of interviewees as essentially passive individuals;
- its reduction of interviewers to a question-asking and rapport-promoting role (Oakley, 1981b, p.36–37).

In the same article Oakley puts forward an alternative model for questioning which is based on grasping the subjectivity of the interview experience, and on mutuality and demystifying 'hygienic' research. She concludes that the personal involvement of the researcher 'is more than dangerous bias – it is the condition under which people come to know each other and to admit others into their lives' (Ibid, p.58). This point of view has been reinforced since the publication of her article, most notably by Stanley and Wise, who state that it is impossible to omit the social persona of the researcher from the research process (1983, p.162).

These considerations are essential when applying the interview mode within the process of change. The researcher as a member of the management structure either has to build on pre-existing relationships, or engage in relationships which will endure beyond the interview episode. Whichever way, there is no denying the existence of the relational aspects of the research encounter. One can draw parallels with the analysis that organizations have an informal structure in which parties maintain social order through diplomacy, bargaining, controlling information, developing different forms of co-operation and so on, and thus create a negotiated order (Strauss *et al.*, 1963). Awareness of negotiation sets the agenda for the interviews, and determines its nature as an exchange, as a formulation of emerging perceptions and assessing the impact of the process of change.

All the interviews took the form of loosely structured thematic discussions aimed at soliciting the respondent's perceptions of the social system and its workings. Thus, a broad spectrum of staff, clients and relatives were asked about the following themes:

1. How they viewed the present service: its operation, management, communication, opportunities etc.
2. How they would like to see the service developing: philosophies, resources, relationships etc.
3. How change could come about and should be managed.

Through discussion of these themes the frames of reference of the various actors in the process of change could be analysed and placed against the background of the proposed structural changes to general management (ward management instead of professional based management). Very importantly, understanding of the perceptions of all the parties involved could not only redirect the change, but also serve as a checking mechanism on the total strategic process.

The second stage of the research consisted of group interviews with selected staff such as CPNs, OTs, social workers, psychologists and a number of managers such as District Heads, Social Services and FPC Senior Officers. The same themes and format as in the individual interviews were followed.

In order to understand the sequence of events one has to realize that the DNS had started to discuss preliminary ideas for the restructuring of the service with Nursing Officers, Charge Nurses and Sisters, the Psychiatric Division, District Heads and trade unions. A considerable amount of antagonism was building up against his plans to streamline the service into three main subunits, covering the acute service, the elderly service and the community, and the devolution of responsibility to ward level.

At the same time the MHR started work with staff groups and Charge

Nurses and Sisters in drawing up personal development plans in line with the proposed management changes. Staff had individual interviews with the DNS and MHR to formulate their needs and translate them into long-term plans for training and development.

The research endeavour slotted into these two parallel activities in providing a different, but complementary perspective on the total process of change. Both individual and group interpretations were analysed in order to assess the response of the social system as a whole. Emerging new frameworks about the structure of the organizations and new roles and responsibilities were identified and could be utilized within the total strategy. This meant that the research had to be part of a team effort and be consistently fed back to managers in order to act as a steering mechanism.

Questions posed by many researchers in the applied policy field centre around the issue of whether the values of managers (or the people who commission research) can be shared by the researcher and require 'value accountability' (Wenger, 1987). In the context of the researcher being part of the management team adherence to the values or mission of the organisation is unavoidable if the research is intended to act as a catalyst for change (Ong, 1989). By the same token, the research endeavour has to be clearly delineated as a scientific exercise, negotiated as a relatively independent activity from the management of change itself. For example, the normal convention of confidentiality was adhered to and thus information given to the MRD was considered to fall under that heading.

In the interviews the MRD was asked questions about the aims and objectives of the managers, and what evidence could be given to prove that this time they were really taking staff's ideas into account. A multitude of methods were proposed including daily visits to the ward by the DNS, open access for individual members of staff, new opportunities for staff development and training, more resources, regular meetings with and without union presence, etc. Without a clear structure of devolved decision-making most of the suggestions remained in an organizational vacuum, and staff had to first accept the creation of an institutional framework which allowed their involvement to grow and develop.

The main feedback mechanism used in the research was through providing regular verbal and written reports. Thus, the results of the observation and questioning methods led to the publication of a paper on the future of rehabilitation services within the Mental Health Unit, explicitly reflecting the results of the research. All respondents could see how their ideas were incorporated into the paper as their contribution was publicly acknowledged. In this way, the research served as a mechanism to unblock ineffective organizational communication channels.

   The document explicitly supported the philosophy of care formulated by the managers and elaborated on that both by using the literature review to examine the scientific state of the art, and translating the research data within the overall framework of analysis. In this way, the merging of the management values and research findings could be accomplished, moving the process of change a step further.

Feeding, directing and sustaining change

The publication of the paper on rehabilitation was followed up with a series of meetings with staff, informal discussions with clients and relatives, and invitations to formally respond, e.g. to MIND. The MRD conducted the meetings within the overall programme of consultation about the changes in the Unit. Thus, three processes took place alongside each other which were mutually reinforcing. Firstly, research oriented discussions, focusing on developing frameworks and models of care whilst also being concerned with the process of change itself. Secondly, management oriented discussions addressing structural and organizational issues. The third strand was the activity generated by the MHR in the field of staff development which underlined the principle of valuing staff. The three elements of the process of change were brought together in regular feedback sessions between the managers involved and the UGM in order to check progress and maintain consistency and coherence (Figure 4.1).

   First, the MRD arranged meetings with separate staff groups which centred around the rehabilitation paper and the principles contained therein. It was important to enable staff to formulate a philosophy

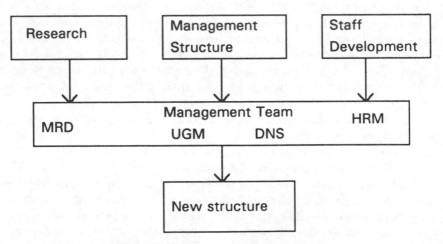

Figure 4.1 Communication structure

establishing a coherent vision of the service as a whole, from prevention to treatment and recovery. Individual assessment of need through care management and flexible service responses were highlighted as key aspects of a good quality service – foreshadowing the ideas of 'Caring for People' (DoH, 1989a). Together with staff, ideas about the 'mission' of the organization could be crystallized and serve as a basis for further work.

Second, strategic discussions focused on the new management arrangements where ward managers would carry 24-hour responsibility for their ward. They would become budget holders and, as such, decision-making was to be devolved to ward level. Staff establishment was determined for each ward according to client needs and the division between day and night was abolished. This structural change created a climate in which ideas such as multidisciplinary teamwork were developed and tested in the various individual and group forums.

Closely related to the change in management roles was the realization that there were more Charge Nurses and Sisters in post than Ward Manager jobs on offer. As with most re-organizations aimed at streamlining, a 'slimmer' top needed to emerge. For each Charge Nurse and Sister this meant a two-fold personal uncertainty: firstly, would there be a job for me at an equivalent level?; secondly, can I deploy my professional skills in a satisfying manner?

This group of staff exhibited the type of response illustrated in other studies (Isabella, 1990): middle managers often feel most vulnerable because they lack the overall picture that top managers have, and in comparison with junior staff they miss the direct hands-on contact with users which allows a sense of self-confidence about the need for their skills. The role of the middle manager is most prone to redefinition in this type of reorganization, resulting in high levels of anxiety and resistance to change in this staff group.

The strategies to redefine change into a positive force and to feed and maintain the process were tailored to the different professional groups in order to respond to their varying perceptions and needs. The dominant influence of the psychiatrists could not be underestimated, and the research approach was crucially important in enlisting their support for the organizational changes. The reliance on scientific literature and original research into the local situation contributed to their confidence in the new management style, based on rigorous examination of problems and prospects. The personal feedback of research results to those psychiatrists interested in the scientific endeavour helped to transmit ideas into the consultants' community, even if direct access to the group as a whole and to their divisional meetings was limited.

The research supported the managerial actions of directly engaging in a dialogue with the psychiatrists most interested in rehabilitation. They were drawn into policy by helping to shape new service developments with managers. Also, regular meetings between the UGM and the Chairperson of the Division helped to iron out differences and to clarify the direction of change.

The issue that caused most concern to the psychiatrists was the accessibility to other professionals, and who would have power over the deployment of personnel. Despite the Griffiths 1983 changes, de facto power over the use of skills of nurses, OTs and psychologists (and to a lesser degree social workers) was in the hands of consultant psychiatrists. Creating a ward management structure would seriously challenge this situation, and psychiatrists would have to negotiate with managers about the use of staff.

The strategies for responding to the nurses were various, but most carefully worked out for the Charge Nurses and Sisters as they were the key opinion makers. The managerial response centred around communication through a series of meetings with the group of senior nurses to discuss a range of issues relating to the organizational change and professional roles. A separate set of meetings took place with trade unions concerned with terms and conditions of service.

Third, the research endeavour supported managerial activities which used dialogue and emphasized staff development. Research was the tangible expression of the new approach to involving staff in developing the service. Through continuous discussion, exchanging ideas about the philosophical and strategic direction of the organization, contrasting those ideas with other research and practice and translating them into an organizational structure capable of consolidating the bottom-up approach, the research confirmed the process of change. Individual members of staff expressed their thoughts in the knowledge that they could make a valuable contribution to the debate, and often saw their ideas validated by others – colleagues or researchers – or incorporated into the new structure.

The research activity served as the feeding mechanism for change: it reflected on the past and present, and continually checked whether the process of change moved towards achieving the agreed aims and objectives. In this sense, the research became an evaluative tool (Lincoln and Guba, 1985) and helped to keep the process 'transparent', thus allowing a measure of control for the participants, both in terms of input and in the application of findings.

Summarized, ethnography as a diagnosis can be an important management tool. Skills in observing organizational interactions and open-ended interviewing are essential requirements for executing this type of project. Furthermore, within the setting of agreed aims and objectives, the research endeavour itself needs to be clearly identified as a separate activity from management in order to maintain credibility. The examination of processes, roles and relationships has to be done 'from within' which makes the role of the researcher somewhat different from that of the traditional detached observer. Although ethnography does not attempt to modify behaviour, its insights into the subjectivity of individuals and organizations can be used within the management of change. Therefore, the researcher becomes more directly accountable for the accuracy and usefulness of the findings. Yet, the implementation of findings has to remain the responsibility of managers, otherwise the researcher's scientific status, which implies relative independence, will be compromised.

CASE 2   UNDERSTANDING USERS' HEALTH CARE NEEDS

The separation of purchasers of health care from those who provide services has pushed the issue of needs assessment centre stage. An important aspect is assessing the needs for specific services, which can rely on professionally based definitions of need, i.e. normative and/or comparative need, or draw on users' own description of need, that is, their felt and/or expressed needs (Bradshaw, 1972). It is important to understand the nature of these definitions, which are derived from different frames of reference, and examine whether and how they converge or diverge. Only comparison can establish a pattern of service needs that is capable of addressing the experiential aspects of disease, and match these with professional capabilities.

Community nursing services

The publication of 'Caring for People' (DoH, 1989a) represents a culmination of the debate about the shift from institutional to community care. One of the key issues emerging in this debate is the relationship between the formal and so-called informal sector of care. Researchers in the social policy field have focused on the nature and costs of caring in the community (Finch and Groves, 1983; Parker, 1990), and demonstrated that increasingly the burden of care is shifting onto the shoulders of those looking after dependent relatives and friends. The growing importance of the informal sector has implications for the professionals in the statutory sector, in that they have to negotiate their role and responsibilities within this delicate network of support. One important group affected by this process are community nurses (Badger *et al.*, 1988; Ong, 1991), and this case study focuses on their service.

In the last two decades nursing has developed as a discrete discipline drawing on a scientific body of knowledge. This is best exemplified in the emergence of nursing models (Orem, 1980; Roper *et al.*, 1980; Roy and Roberts, 1981) which are firmly based on the professional assessment of need. Yet, the community nursing context is the arena *par excellence* where a dialogue between professional and user is an essential element in the formulation of care needs. Furthermore, the social context of the user often includes carers, who not only have a distinct perspective on users' needs but also have needs of their own, illustrated by a growing body of literature (Glendinning, 1986; Ayer and Alaszewski, 1986; Green, 1988; Land, 1991).

Considering the above complexity, community nurses have to be able to answer a number of questions which can distinguish between how users and carers define their needs, how they compare with professional assessments, and finally, what responses community nurses can offer. An in-depth analysis of the first question forms the starting point for the formulation of managerial responses, which can be matched with available resources.

Ethnography in defining care needs

An important methodological device in ethnography is the interview, which most usually takes the form of a thematic conversation. The main purpose of the interview is to uncover people's perceptions and experiences. In the case of studying health care needs, an understanding has to be built up about the way health and illness are framed by cultural notions. For example, Finch (1989) has demonstrated how obligations within families are culturally bounded and define the norms guiding social behaviour.

The objective for the study on community nursing was to formulate the key concerns that users and carers expressed in defining their nursing needs, and the role of community nurses in meeting those needs. Painting the contextual background of illness in modern society served to understand the experiences and reasoning of users, but only in order to distil a list of issues. These issues were intended to feed into an analysis of current community nursing in order to inform managers of the best 'fit' between perceived needs and service response. In short, the ethnographic method was deployed primarily to ensure that issues emerged from the users' and carers' own experiential accounts.

The research, therefore, was designed as a multistage project. Firstly, in collaboration with a representative group of community nurses, the researcher delineated the broad themes for the interviews, starting with a historical account of the person's illness, to understanding its impact on their lives. This could be followed by a description of needs, and health care needs specifically, and end with a discussion of the expectations and role of community nurses in meeting those needs.

Secondly, the data gathering was carried out in a series of semi-structured interviews which were conducted as a guided conversation, and fully tape recorded and transcribed. The analysis was two-fold: to generate concepts and to translate those into a list of key concerns.

Thirdly, this list was discussed with community nurses and managers in order to formulate organizational responses, and to feed into a separate activity analysis.

Sampling

The purpose of the study could be defined as exploratory in its search for concepts. This also meant that the study intended to generalize from the small case study. Generalization in qualitative research has been a contentious area, because it builds on different assumptions than quantitative research, where probability is a key concept. Sampling in quantitative research tends to be designed in such a way that the selection of cases from the study population depends upon chance alone, and not upon the researcher's judgement. Probability samples are samples in which each case has a known – but not necessarily equal – chance of being selected.

Qualitative research focuses on processes and perceptions, and aims in its construction of 'social structure' to generate universals and principles from particular social phenomena (Stanley, 1990). In the concrete study, the specific social phenomenon of health care within a community setting was to generate insights about the experience of illness, the definitions of need and the division of labour between formal and informal care. The findings were intended to form the basis for decisions about the structure and nature of one particular form of care provision, i.e. community nursing.

Precisely because of its exploratory nature sampling required a carefully constructed approach. Non-random sampling was most appropriate in this situation, and more specifically, a form of conceptual sampling was chosen. Thus, the researcher discussed with the group of community nurses the descriptive characteristics of the population under study. Three key variables emerged:

1. the caring environment, i.e. whether a client had carer support, and in which form;
2. the socio-geographical context: four distinctly different locations could be identified;
3. clinical condition and specific nursing procedures.

A three-dimensional matrix was constructed producing 176 cells. Of course, it was technically impossible to conduct that number of in-depth interviews, and with the additional carers. Instead, from this matrix, ten cases were selected representing the agreed key characteristics. The health care needs of the study population could be formulated from in-depth coverage of those cases. The selection offered scope to examine similarities and differences between the cases, thus allowing for testing explanations against contrasting evidence. With this approach generaliz-able concepts are constructed not through randomization, but through focused sampling against an explicit set of criteria (Mitchell, 1983).

An important feature of ethnography is that it demonstrates that the researcher has 'been there' (Geertz in Stanley, 1990). Whether the people studied feel that ethnographic description represent their experiences requires careful checking, and the process of being researched has been candidly exposed in some texts (Kendall and Dodson, 1990). In the community nursing study all interviewees received the transcribed copy for approval, and could amend the text if they wished to do so.

The experience of illness

Locker (1981) has argued that the social aspects of illness can be understood within a framework which dichotomizes order and disorder. Then, illness can be defined as a disturbance in a person's social and physical functioning. This notion clearly emerges in discussing the impact of chronic illness, where, for example, one lady labels her MS (multiple sclerosis) as 'the beginning and ending of the word 'mess'. The physical self and her trust in her body has been shattered, causing the rest of her life to be adversely affected. This process demonstrates the interplay between person, body and ailment in an individual within the context of social interaction (Stacey, 1988).

The impact of disease on self-conception has been studied through the concept of patient career. People with chronic illness (who constitute a large part of community nurses' caseloads) have been forced to redefine their identity, and negotiate different relationships with their own social networks and with professionals. This negotiation is determined by factors such as the nature and stage of the disease, types of treatment, social circumstances, professional approaches, etc. Most importantly, it centres around the distribution of power and control (Waitzkin and Stoeckle, 1972).

The two theoretical notions of disease as disorder and patient career are important when examining the users' self-perceptions and their needs. The first group of clients saw their personhood to be untouched by disease. They considered their personal identity separate from their disease, and consequently bracketed off nursing care needs from the rest of their lives. For them community nurses had a well-defined task to accomplish by providing support so that they could lead a normal life. This outlook did not depend on the severity of the disease.

The second group regarded the disease as a discrete episode, and placed boundaries as to professional involvement and help. They accepted that the disease had an impact on their life, but defined the territories where this was acceptable. In consequence, the areas where nursing care was required were also carefully delineated.

The majority of clients in the study, however, did not distinguish between physical, social and psychological aspects of illness. They invited nurses to provide holistic care, and considered the totality of their situation as an appropriate terrain for professional involvement. The dominant nursing philosophy of dealing with the whole person, within their social context, appeared to match client expectations.

The experience of caring

The growing body of knowledge about caring has demonstrated its importance within the social policy context. Twigg *et al.* (1990) and Twigg and Atkin (1990) argue that caring is socially constructed, and as a result has to be understood within its wider social context. They develop a typology of carers which describes their self-identities, either as being engulfed by the caring role, as being in a symbiotic relationship with the cared for or as boundary setters, distinguishing their own needs from those of the cared for.

Furthermore, they discuss the different relationships carers and professionals can engage in: carers can be seen as co-workers or as (taken for granted) resources. The delicate interplay of self-definition and professional perceptions of the caring role produces a series of different interactions, and subsequent roles for community nursing. Managers need to understand the origin and nature of these complexities in order to explain the pattern of needs and demands presented to them, and to question professional needs assessment.

The key issues

From the contextual analysis of the experiences of illness and caring a set of key issues could be extracted which served as focal points for a review of community nursing services. The first set of issues related to the organization of work. Dependability and punctuality were considered essential by both carers and users because they wanted to maintain a sense of regularity and control over their lives. Yet, this was contradictory to their demand for flexibility of response, which meant that they wanted access to professional help outside appointed times. But flexibility had as its main cost the loss of predictability.

The content of care was judged in terms of the quality of communications between nurses, i.e. whether they had sufficient knowledge about users' needs when taking over care from each other. Also, continuity of care, in particular between different care settings, was seen as an important indicator.

Taken together, these issues set the agenda for a comparative approach to the organizational review. Two response systems were to be evaluated against each other, one focusing on dependability, and the other focusing on flexibility. After an agreed pilot period opinions of users and carers would be sampled about the effectiveness of each system. Simultaneously, managers reviewed communications between and within teams as well as communications between hospital, GPs and other community based professionals and the community nursing service.

Health workers have increasingly had to accept user feedback on the form and context of service provision, but have been reluctant to solicit and value feedback on the content of their service. This point of view is hard to sustain when dealing with experienced users, such as most community nursing patients. They have dealt with a number of professionals during their patient career, and have built up a body of knowledge which enables them to judge professional competence. Thus, many users prioritized the technical expertise of nurses before other skills such as providing advice and displaying good interpersonal skills. Interestingly, most users made a distinction between tasks that required trained or untrained staff.

With the advent of clinical audit the above insights place the users centre stage. Quality of technical aspects of care can be judged by those receiving the service, and user-defined indicators should be included in audit. This issue has to be taken on board by managers, and the results from ethnographic research can provide them with the ingredients for creating a multifaceted audit system.

Finally, the dominant nursing philosophy of providing holistic care was only acceptable to those users who did not bracket off their disease from the totality of their life. The people who did not consider their disease to impact on their self identity, or those who limited it to a specific area of their life, considered holistic nursing intrusive. At the same time, almost all users and carers saw a concern for carers' health and well-being as an integral part of the nursing task. This contradiction could not be managed at the level of the client population, and required a flexible adaptation of the philosophy at the individual level.

Managers and community nurses had to reflect on current practice, and examine the appropriateness of applying particular nursing models to the home care context. The complex interplay of user and carer needs pointed unambiguously in the direction of multidisciplinary and multi-agency working, and as such provided an excellent case for putting *Caring for People* principles into practice. Rather than relying on professional dogma, the analysis of need and subsequent flexible response opened up new avenues for matching assessment and resource deployment more accurately.

In summary, the ethnographic study of community nursing revealed a complex picture of need, related to a variety of self-perceptions and experiences of illness. It is important for providers to understand this cultural context in order to be able to grasp the essence of felt and expressed needs of users and their carers. An analysis of specific health care needs can then be grounded in in-depth knowledge of the nature and circumstances of disease. Service responses can be better targeted, and skills and resources deployed accordingly.

CONCLUSION

Ethnography in health service management can be most productively applied if it takes the form of insightful description, i.e. if it presents phenomena in new and revealing ways (Hammersley, 1990). Goffman's work on 'total institutions' is an eminent example of this type of ethnography (Goffman, 1961) which has influenced the thinking of health and social service managers up to the present day.

Ethnography can also describe events and relationships in context, and precisely because of this contextualization ethnography can be explanatory. For example, the work on the experience of carers within western society, with its particular division of labour and norms about familial obligations, provides an explanation of why care in the community tends to be predominantly care by women in the community (Dalley, 1988). This is an important consideration for managers when planning and targeting services.

Ethnography as a first stage for the development of theory or as the application of theory tends to have more academic than managerial relevance, but certain theoretical insights can, of course, guide the research process. Furthermore, methodological considerations can be transposed from the academic to the health service setting, and the discussion on sampling has been one example. The unique contribution of ethnography to health service management is that it provides an understanding from within, that is, ethnography attempts to understand the world from the perspective of the people who are the subject of research. It is capable of reflecting on the reasoning and feelings of the recipients of health services, and gaining insights in 'what it feels like' to be a user. This is crucially important if services are to become more responsive to people's needs.

Secondly, ethnography is flexible, and can study process. As such it is eminently suitable for describing and monitoring change. Managers require this processual evidence if they are to lead organizations in turbulence, because it allows them to keep 'a finger on the pulse', and anticipate and steer the direction of a service that is sensitive to its staff and its users.

Chapter Five

Participatory and action research models

INTRODUCTION

With the introduction of general management, and reinforced by recent government publications such as *Working for Patients* (DoH, 1989b), *Caring for People* (DoH, 1989a), *The Health of the Nation* (DoH, 1992) and *The Patient's Charter* (1991b), the ascendancy of the service user in health care policy has been secured. At the same time, the definition of users and their role in health service planning and provision has been obscured. Instead, emphasis is placed on setting targets, without elaboration of their philosophical and theoretical underpinning. As a result, policy and management in relation to service users move in a conceptual vacuum, and methodologies for involving users appear to be ad hoc and untested.

This chapter will explore the different ways in which users can be conceptualized, and their implications for the definition of participation. Reference will be made to the historical origins of user participation, and the various interpretations employed within health strategies. Different methodologies will be discussed, which offer systematic approaches to encouraging user participation in planning services. Nationally, the NHS Management Executive launched in 1992 an initiative called *Local Voices: The Views of Local People in Purchasing for Health* which explicitly states that health authorities should engage in a dialogue with local people on the assumption that their views are valued and may influence purchasing intentions. Although the principle of community participation appears to have been endorsed, many conceptual and research issues remain to be clarified.

DEFINING USERS

Policy documents tend to be vague about definitions, and the key documents relating to the 1989 NHS reorganizations hardly address the conundrum of who the users are. The immediate questions to be raised are whether users are those people who are receiving health care themselves: are they people who look after dependents who are receiving care, e.g. parents of young children, are they people who are on waiting lists, are they people who have undetected, unmet needs, etc.?

Apart from this question of categorizing the different types of users into indirect, direct and potential, there is a more conceptual distinction about how users are viewed: as consumers or as participants in the planning, delivery and evaluation of health care. We will elaborate on this distinction as it will necessitate very different relationships with managers, and determine the research agenda in opposite directions.

The user as consumer

The policy framework outlined in *The Health of the Nation* (DoH, 1992) is circumscribed by two key concerns: to maximize the efficiency or output of the NHS, and to change the behaviour of individuals (Radical Statistics Group, 1991). A logical corollary is to focus on the contribution that health services and individual behaviours are making to health maintenance. From this perspective users are seen as potential contributors, either by participating in health service activities – for example, the Patient's Charter actively encourages people to become donors or volunteers – or by providing feedback as a consumer of services.

The user as consumer model draws its inspiration directly from the business world. Research into the changing population is crucially important in order to deduct from demographic shifts the future patterns of needs. Thus, an understanding of groups of people and their social and cultural characteristics forms the basis on which the consumer model is built. But, the philosophical core of the model is the notion of choice: consumers make decisions about whether, where and how to use health care.

Within this paradigm health care does not essentially differ from other consumer goods.

This approach is grounded in the reality that the health service provides a diverse range of services which are not urgent, and therefore, potential choice can be exercised about the uptake of those services. It can be argued that good health is desirable but not always an absolute priority, therefore creating space for choice – as smoking, drinking and eating behaviour testify (Green in Devlin *et al.*, 1990). Blaxter (1990) has pointed out that the choice of lifestyle is a contentious area of debate. She argues that both social and economic circumstances, and the more voluntary aspects of lifestyle, are associated with health, but the question remains as to which is the most important. Evidence exists to support either, and decisions based on the social or the individual oriented perspective lead to very different perceptions of users.

The central precondition for exercising choice is access to information. The holders of information are those who deliver the services: medical, nursing and paramedical personnel have intimate knowledge about the technical and clinical aspects, whilst the managers have knowledge about the organization and structure. Much has been written about the professionals' perceptions of esoteric knowledge, and their inability to impart information to the user (Comaroff, 1976; McIntosh, 1977). Managers within a business environment have used information to shape the views of consumers, but health service managers have paid relatively little attention to their relationship to users until the advent of general management.

This tendency has been reinforced by the new agenda which focuses attention on imparting information to users in order for them to make choices. In the purchaser–provider division various users can be targeted: 'proxy' users such as GP fundholders and commissioning authorities or the actual users and their carers. Whatever the relationship with the user, be it direct or indirect, professionals and managers have to work closely together in order to offer a package of information that attracts business. Thus, the content and focus of information alters fundamentally in that clinical knowledge has to be combined with information about the process of delivery, expected outcomes and cost-effectiveness. As such, the barriers of esoteric scientific knowledge have to be broken down. Equally, the veil has to be lifted from the structural issues such as priority setting, the organization of care, accountability and resource allocation. The new agenda has opened up arenas that were hitherto hidden from view, and it has blurred disciplinary boundaries, notably between clinical/professional and managerial information. As a result, there has to be joint responsibility between managers and professionals about the content and form of information giving.

Potentially this new direction allows greater insight on the part of the users. There are two problems, however. Firstly, information is still largely controlled by the stake holders, and this determines the nature and shape of the information released. Secondly, information is framed within the context of 'limited competition', and as such is not necessarily relevant to direct users who judge information against their personal needs. Much information now collected and disseminated is not geared towards those who actually use health care themselves, but towards the professional and managerial 'proxies' who are considered to be capable of defining user need in order to commission the right balance of services.

Underlying the whole approach to information is the assumption that all users can make a choice. It is obvious that choice is contextualized by social and cultural circumstances, and the debate about whether health behaviour is an individual decision or a structurally bounded one is an illustration *par excellence* (RUHBC, 1989). Thus, choice is not a unitary concept, and there are large groups of users who cannot exercise choice because they are limited by psychological, social, cultural or economic factors. It is important to address this issue of differential empowerment if users are to be given equal access to information and choice.

Notwithstanding all the complexities of imparting information and ensuring that users can make choices, the model of the user as consumer centres around the notion that people consciously select health care and that they have expectations against which outcomes can be measured. It is therefore logical to see customer satisfaction surveys as the main method for testing this hypothesis. The new providers are particularly keen to pursue this as they are searching for tools that can help them test their market and develop their products (Baker, 1991).

Customer satisfaction surveys tend to formulate hypotheses which are derived from organizational values, and are often phrased as absolutes. For example, patients want friendly and courteous staff, want pleasant surroundings, do not want to wait longer than 15 minutes. Health care is broken down into quantifiable entities, which are assumed to make up the whole and allow some assessment about the quality of the service (see The Patient's Charter, DoH, 1991). Of course, the main limitation is that these elements can only be seen as indicators of something larger that has both quantitative and qualitative characteristics. Precisely because health care is a service, and therefore relies on human interaction, quantification of customer satisfaction becomes a very tricky exercise.

Another important point is that satisfaction is a relative indicator and has to be evaluated against alternative choices that could have been made. Theoretically the 1989 reorganization widens the menu of alternatives for users, but in reality choices are limited because other non-health costs, such as longer travelling times, are a deterrent for exercising free choice. Thus, satisfaction will largely remain bounded by the range of services offered in a particular locality, hospital or district, and patient satisfaction has to be evaluated within those limits.

The user as consumer model demands a limited contribution from users in that they give feedback on what policy makers, managers and clinicians offer. Furthermore, their involvement is focused on health service provision, and not on health policy or strategy. Thus, the user as consumer remains passive and consequently research methodologies aim to reflect consumer satisfaction, using market research tools rather than user preference, which demand a qualitative and conceptual approach.

The user as participant

The model that defines the user as a participant in the planning and delivery of health care has a number of theoretical foundations. At a global level the United Nations promoted a community development approach aimed at instigating change from within communities. In the 1960s the notion of communities as homogeneous units was overturned with the emergence of diverse movements such as women's liberation, black and ethnic minorities' rights, peace and students' movements. The concept of oppression became central in the analyses of these groups and the work of Paulo Freire (1972), who advocated consciousness-raising through revolutionary community education, became influential.

These strands of thinking filtered through in health care philosophies, and the social developments in the People's Republic of China were an important catalyst. This country had made dramatic strides in improving the population's health through far-reaching public health and community development applications (Horn, 1969; Sidel and Sidel,1983). At the other end of the world the Lalonde report (1974) published in Canada set out new principles for a public health movement grounded in community diagnosis. These ideas from different corners of the globe pointed towards the need for an approach to health policy and planning which placed communities and users centre stage.

The WHO Health for All philosophy synthesized these ideas into a coherent framework (WHO, 1981). It emphasizes understanding health needs within a political context shaped by social and economic forces. People's health is multidimensional and the involvement of communities in determining the input of statutory organizations is crucial for a successful interplay between all the different factors which determine health. The WHO European targets (WHO, 1985) are based on the same notion of the empowered user of health services and are central to the debate about the relationship between users and managers.

From another perspective particular client groups have questioned the notion of the user as (passive) consumer of services. The clearest example is provided by the case of pregnant women who do not fall within the disease category. Moreover, the professionals assisting women in childbirth have to rely on the active participation of the client in order to achieve a successful outcome. This situation presents professionals and managers with a paradox (Oakley, 1981). Control over the process and outcome has, of necessity, to be shared with the client and poses fundamental questions about the role of the user.

The theoretical analysis of this tension and the active campaigning of women for a service which recognizes the important role of the user has opened up the possibilities of real client involvement in planning and delivery. This particular struggle was supported by some midwives who felt that they were being deskilled because of the medical interventionist domination of obstetrics (Kirkham, 1986; Renfrew and McCandlish, 1992)). Tangible results such as broadening the choices for how and where to deliver (falling short of expanding home deliveries) can be pinpointed.

The above two strands of user involvement illustrate two different points of departure: the first one conceptualizes the user as a social being who perceives a totality of need of which health needs are one aspect. The main entrance point for making services sensitive to users' needs is seen to lie in changing overall health policy and planning. The second one defines the user as a consumer of a specific service who wants to gear that service to her or his individual need through changing its structure and character. These two perspectives utilize different research tools in order to pursue different strategies. The first one elaborates on a community development approach, whilst the latter builds on an advocacy and feedback model.

CREATING RELATIONSHIPS THROUGH COMMUNITY DEVELOPMENT

The introduction of general management initiated the push for devolution of power and decision-making down the National Health Service, which provided the impetus for 'going local'. Many community units, delivering primary health care such as nursing, paramedical, medical and dental services, created new management structures reflecting this trend (Dalley, 1987; Ong, 1989). With the decentralization accountability to the local community became a real possibility as the management and planning processes took place closer to the user, and were potentially more visible. Managers began to seriously think about the role of the user in planning and evaluating health care.

Units which operated with an explicit philosophy of care based on the HFA principles viewed user participation as intrinsically linked with the issue of equity (Rifkin et al., 1988). Health care is ultimately aimed at giving people equal opportunities to achieve optimal health, and within a context of continuing inequality (Townsend, 1990) resources have to be distributed unequally. This necessitates the assessment of need and the setting of priorities; in short, a national health strategy should define the parameters (DoH, 1992; Jacobson, et al., 1991).

The NHS changes proposed in 1989 offer real opportunities to focus on communities as districts, FHSAs and GP fundholders are funded to commission services directly related to the size and the characteristics of the population they serve. Knowledge of communities' needs and preferences becomes a fundamental requirement for effective and efficient commissioning. Yet, the ways in which communication with communities can be established are often unclear to many commissioning agencies. Current medical and managerial dominance in priority setting does not take account of the perceptions of users, and this discrepancy has often led to an underutilization of services, for example, the failure of many child immunization programmes. The HFA framework offers a different perspective and takes as its starting point the concept that health improves through community participation, and that broad participation builds on a wide range of activities and involvement of many different community groups (Rifkin *et al.*, 1988).

Two issues need clarification. Firstly, there are various levels of participation and Maxwell (1984) distinguishes five levels: consumer protection – which is a minimum demand; public consultation; openness of managerial decision-making; full participation, with communities sharing in the process of health policy making; and lastly, a radical shift in the balance of power away from those providing the services to those who use them. There are no clear dividing lines between the various levels, and we see openness of managerial decision-making as a precondition for moving to the latter two levels. In our discussion we will focus precisely on that dynamic.

Secondly, describing a community is a particularly tricky problem (Hillery, 1955; Bell and Newby, 1971; Pahl, 1984). It can be defined as a geographical entity, for example, a housing estate; it can be a cultural entity, such as Travellers; it can be a client group, such as people with physical disabilities – yet these groupings are deficient in that they overlap or are still too gross to take account of intricate differences. The question is how fine distinctions have to be for planning, or whether locally based services have sufficient flexibility to re-adjust service delivery on the ground and thus some broad generalizations could encompass the key priorities.

The present political context which views citizens as individual consumers poses particular dilemmas for community development, which has tended to base its practice on the model of conflict between the individual and the state. Instead, Hawker (1989) states that participation in the management, development and implementation of systems provided under a representative democracy is a complex business and that the distribution of power lies at the heart of the debate. Precisely because of the intricacy and sheer size of the NHS managers need a more formalized relationship with users and the balance of power has to be carefully negotiated.

An important example of research which starts by asking local people and workers what they think, need and want in relation to health policy and provision is the West Lambeth study on Clapham, London (Dun, 1989a). A large community health survey was undertaken as part of the PATCH (Primary Action Towards Community Health) pilot project. It was geographically based and utilized 'lay', locally recruited, community health workers who facilitated and organized local community health action.

The study intended to enable people to redefine health and health needs, in order that the results would influence planners and policy makers. It used a 'bottom-up' approach, and emphasized the necessity of including lay perspectives in formulating a complete picture of health. It also aimed to identify patterns of services needed, and to define actions to redress health inequities.

Grassroots workers were also interviewed, as they often feel that they have little influence in the planning process. The overall approach was multisectoral, in line with the WHO definition of health as a totality.

The methodology was multistaged, starting with qualitative interviews with key informants and staging group discussions, which were to produce the framework for the larger community survey. This survey used open-ended questions to elicit perceptions of health, and from the responses categories were produced which allowed quantitative measurement (Dun, 1989b). The questionnaire aimed to compare and contrast lay with professional perspectives, to identify local problems and to suggest local solutions.

In total, four samples were studied: health workers, social services workers, voluntary sector and a 1% general household quota sample. Following the analysis a list of general and specific recommendations was formulated, specifically geared towards the Health Authority, but also directed at the Family Health Services Authority, Local Authority and voluntary sector. The main thrust was for managers to 'go local'. Finally, recommendations were formulated directly aimed at citizens and consumers, which stressed the importance of their continued participation in policy and planning.

The second example comes from Dallam, Warrington, where a multisectoral group (Health Authority, Local Authority, voluntary sector and Community Health Council) undertook a health project to define areas where the community considered help was needed (Snee, 1991). It was realized that community priorities were not necessarily the same as those of statutory/voluntary agencies, but the project was considered a point of departure for constructive dialogue between the two parties.

Community involvement in the project was secured through a steering group, consisting of seven people from the local community who participated as interested individuals, and four workers from different agencies. The project was based on the idea of partnership, with local people having the final say over the direction of the project. Founded in the HFA2000 philosophy, a community health approach was used, defined as 'a process whereby a community defines its own needs and organises to meet these needs, where appropriate, and to make them known to the service providers in order to bring about change' (Snee, 1991, p.5).

A questionnaire, to be administered in the community, was devised based on the ideas of the steering group, discussions with different agencies and consultations with experts in methodology, epidemiology and community surveys (notably two residents from Moyard, Belfast, on which this project was modelled). The questionnaire served as a scientific instrument, and as a tool for stimulating collective action among local people. It went through several redrafting stages in which input from residents was crucial.

Every household (617) in the area received a questionnaire, which was distributed by local residents. The questionnaire was primarily for self-completion, but six members of the steering group were trained in interview procedures to help respondents who were unable to fill in the questionnaire themselves. The collection of the questionnaire was, again, done door to door, and a 70% response rate was secured. The whole exercise was backed up by a publicity drive and a raffle.

The outcome of the Dallam project was a specific list of recommendations, rather than to demonstrate 'theory-in-practice' of community development. It provided a lesson in valuing and fostering the talents and commitments of 'ordinary' people, and in demonstrating the changes needed in the education and understanding of agency professionals and government bodies (Snee, 1991, p.51). The report of the study was presented as the start for the development of an action plan between the people of Dallam and the agencies who serve the area.

THE CASE STUDY: RAPID APPRAISAL IN URBAN DEPRIVED COMMUNITIES

Traditional community development approaches aimed at empowerment of the community have tended to oversimplify the process of decision-making (Croft and Beresford, 1990) and methodologies which tackle the complex relationship between managers – and professionals – and users have to be developed. The case study focuses on an alternative application of community development research aimed at clarifying and modifying the relationship between managers and users.

There has been considerable opposition to community development approaches in health as they are considered to deal primarily with raising political consciousness rather than with the delivery of 'objective' data about the state of health of a community (Stewart-Brown and Protheroe, 1988). Managers have often been reluctant about community development approaches because they believe them to be time-consuming and to deliver intangible results. Because they are small scale they frequently fail to make an impact on policy formulation as generalization from the one case is more difficult.

Given these reservations, and the need to create a more direct link between local managers and users, an alternative methodology which can tackle both the logistical and the philosophical problems has to be developed. Essentially community participation needs to be achieved in the following key areas:

- diagnosis;
- decision-taking and priority setting;
- implementation;
- benefiting;
- evaluation (Nichter, 1984; Hawker, 1989).

Rapid Appraisal, a methodology used by social scientists and predominantly applied in developing countries, displays characteristics which are central to participatory research geared towards change:

1. greater speed compared with conventional methods of analysis;
2. working in the 'field';
3. an emphasis on learning directly from local inhabitants;
4. a semi-structured, multidisciplinary approach with room for flexibility and innovation;
5. an emphasis on producing timely insights, hypotheses or 'best bets' rather than final truths or fixed recommendations (Conway, 1988).

Annett and Rifkin (1988) have adapted this framework for investigation in the health field, linking it with the HFA philosophy. With the focus on equity they target members of urban environments that are still denied the benefits of the residents of more affluent urban situations. Regarding participation they use 'key informants' both to identify community problems and to contribute to solutions. In keeping with the multisectoral approach they work with resource holders from various (statutory) organizations to carry out the investigations and to formulate a plan of action.

A major tool in collecting data about the totality of the community experience of health, and of individuals within the community, is an 'information profile'. This serves both as a guide to the collection of material, and as the organizing framework for the analysis.

Looking more closely at the various elements of the profile, researchers need to start from an understanding of the demographic composition of the community, its internal informal and formal organization and its capacity to act. From there, factors impinging on the health of a community are socio-ecological and economic, and some insight into the possibilities or barriers to controlling those factors has to be gained in order to assess areas of improvement. The influence of statutory organizations and the benefits their services offer is the next layer of investigation. Quality measures such as accessibility, acceptability and effectiveness can be indicators for change. Finally, placing the whole exercise within the context of national policy regarding inequalities and urban deprivation will show the degree of commitment to the cause of improving health for all.

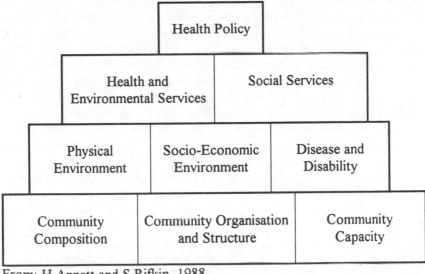

From: H Annett and S Rifkin, 1988

Figure 5.1 Information profile

The Rapid Appraisal methodology offers very specific insights: it can tell *what* the problems in a particular community are, but *not how many* people are affected by those problems. Or, to put it differently, it can tell what the strength of feeling is within a community. Understanding this subjectivity is important because it largely determines how people are acting and utilizing the services provided. For example, the number of people on hard drugs can be relatively small, but their impact on the harmony of a community can be immense. Community resources can become preoccupied with dealing with that problem to the detriment of addressing other issues that affect larger numbers of people, for example the use of minor tranquillizers.

Rapid Appraisal defines a community as a social rather than a geographical entity. This means that understanding of a community has to be generated through the diverse perspectives present in that community. Thus, knowledge is built up on the basis of different 'truths' and information is, therefore, collected from a variety of 'key informants'.

Basically, these key people can be categorized as follows:

- Professionals operating within a given community who can provide a specific and focused perspective, for example teachers, GPs, nurses, social workers.
- Leaders and self-elected leaders who represent particular interests and factions, for example local councillors, a convenor of the neighbourhood watch scheme.
- People who are social focal points, such as shopkeepers.

The information given by these three sets of people provides a complex picture, based on an 'inter-subjective' understanding of community living. It is important to select informants carefully in order to gain contrasting views which assist in testing emerging hypotheses. The most effective approach is snowball sampling, whereby respondents are asked to name others who might be useful and willing to discuss the topic of research.

Rapid Appraisal has two aims: it is a research tool for describing priority needs, and as such focuses on health as a total concept. The multidisciplinary approach involves the communities as current and potential users with managers from statutory organizations (health, social services, education, housing, environmental health, etc.) in the planning process. Participation in decision-making about resource allocation provides the basis for people to give feedback on services: do they satisfy an identified need, and are they delivered in a manner that is acceptable to users? As such, Rapid Appraisal can be a tool for both purchasers and providers.

Secondly, Rapid Appraisal is the starting point for establishing longer term relationships with constituent communities. Needs and preferences are constantly changing, and an ongoing dialogue with communities is an important mechanism for tailoring services to people's needs. Rapid Appraisal can, therefore, be repeated at regular intervals in order to assess progress.

Doing a Rapid Appraisal

Applications in the UK (Ong *et al.*, 1991) have all taken place in urban areas with high levels of deprivation, measured by using Jarman (Jarman, 1983) or similar indicators (Thunhurst, 1985). The process and results from three exercises will be discussed in this section.

Rapid Appraisal is a flexible method, which continues to be developed and can be adapted to local circumstances. Broadly, the following steps have to be carried out:

1. Preparation by a small team of managers (or one individual) aimed to secure participation from a wide range of organizations, i.e. a multidisciplinary and multi-agency approach.
2. A two-day workshop which outlines the principles and scope of the method. The target population has to be chosen on the basis of available secondary data, and organizational knowledge. Key questions and issues to be researched have to be determined, using the information profile framework, and an interview schedule formu-

lated. Furthermore, a first sample of respondents needs to be drawn up.

3. Fieldwork: the collection of secondary data, observations of the neighbourhoods, open-ended interviews with respondents, and generating the snowball sample. Small teams will work together in accomplishing these three tasks, and begin with a preliminary analysis of their data.

4. Half-day workshop to collate all the findings from the subteams, and extract a list of needs as defined by the community (the needs should be ordered, whenever possible, within the categories of the information profile).

5. Research team returns to individual respondents with the request to place all identified needs in priority order (by category).

6. Analysis of priorities (computer assisted or manual), and discussion of the results in a half-day workshop. The team has to prepare for a meeting with the community by formulating proposals for action.

7. Open meeting with respondents and interested members of the community to discuss findings and proposals. This meeting should, if possible, formulate concrete action plans.

8. Establishing ongoing working relationships for evaluation and revision of action plans.

Research skills for this method are limited to ethnographic interviewing (which is offered in basic form in the first workshop) and skills in SPSS if computer assisted analysis is used. Guidance for the overall process will have to be bought in from people experienced in the method, and who are able to direct the workshops.

The first UK based Rapid Appraisal was carried out in Linacre ward, Bootle, on Merseyside (Ong and Humphris, 1990; Ong *et al.*, 1991). This ward suffers from social and economic deprivation such as unemployment, with rates in excess of 20%, with the majority of houses being council-owned, and high levels of pollution from the adjacent freeport (Schoon, 1992). The 1989 Rapid Appraisal results are shown in Table 5.1. The ratings were based on the community's set of priorities. These could be compared with the priorities selected by the research team, which were based predominantly on managerial priorities. A detailed inspection and comparison of the priority ratings was possible, which was considered as very valuable in discussions between the team members and the community.

Action plans resulting from the priority listing have to be clearly delineated in scope and timescale. They also have to secure a contribution from both the community and statutory agencies, and deliver a clear product to be evaluated.

Three action plans were agreed with the community, with the first one

Table 5.1   Linacre ward, 1989. Community priorities

Physical environment	(0.12)**
1. Rubbish in the street	2. 19
2. Poor quality housing	2.69
3. Air pollution	3.19
4. Disposal of syringes in public places	3.38
5. Lack of recreational space	3.56
Disease and disability	(0.07)
1. Depression and anxiety	2.19
2. Drinking, tobacco, tranquillizers, hard drugs	2.34
3. Respiratory problems	2.50
4. Poor diet	2.97
Health services	(0.27)**
1. Lack of overall preventive children's services	2.34
2. GPs appear 'too busy'	2.58
3. Lack of home support after hospital discharge	2.59
4. Lack of well woman services	3.09
5. Lack of chiropody services	4.39
Social services	(0.17)***
1. Information is not readily available	2.00
2. Lack of pre-school facilities	2.13
3. Fear of the power of SSDs to remove children	2.72
4. Home helps are not free of charge	3.16
Socio-economic environment	(0.34)***
1. Unemployment	1.34
2. Financial problems, debt	2.19
3. Environment generally unsafe (e.g. robberies)	2.47
The community's own valuable resources	(0.37)***
1. Strong family support systems	2.13
2. Strong community action groups	2.66
3. 'Bootle identity'	2.95
4. Good local councillors	3.73
5. Support from churches	4.44
6. Community Health Council	5.09

Figures in brackets are Kendall's coefficient of concordance, i.e. a measure of agreement amongst the 'judges' ranks.
* $p<0.05$; ** $p<0.01$; *** $p<0.0001$ (significance levels).

providing support to the Residents' Association in their fight against air pollution from the firms based at the docks. The consultant paediatrician embarked on a study of respiratory illness amongst schoolchildren near the coaldust area, in order to compare their levels with those of six other Merseyside schools. In parallel, a group of students from the Liverpool

School of Tropical Medicine carried out a series of case histories of people with respiratory illness (Baqwa *et al.*, 1990). Evidence from these studies will assist the community to present their case in two court battles to stop the dumping of coaldust.

The second action plan was more time limited because both the Local Authority and Community Unit (Health) provided specific professional help in the setting up of a food co-operative and credit union. The local groups had some training in book-keeping, bulk buying and input from the dietician in food preparation. After this initial start-up support the professionals withdrew to let the groups run the operation themselves.

The third project was to give a mother and toddler group training in detecting and preventing depression. Occupational therapists ran a number of sessions to teach people to help themselves through relaxation exercises. They also instructed people when and where to call for professional help.

These three action plans were to be evaluated after six months, with the Locality Manager (Health) as the key person to monitor the process, and to instigate further meetings and action plans. The first round of projects had been supported and seen through by the original research team, consisting of senior managers. Thus, the objective of tangible action was achieved. However, with the turbulence in many of the organizations the second objective of continuing dialogue was more difficult to attain. The Locality Manager post was taken up by three different people in the space of one year, and most of the original team moved on to other jobs in the same period. This meant that long-term relationships with the community could not be properly established, and the momentum of the Rapid Appraisal could not be maintained.

Learning from this experience, the second Rapid Appraisal was designed to secure continuity. As a result, the composition of the research team was different, and relied more on middle managers from a range of organizations. The community selected had a similar profile to Linacre ward, being a geographically bounded estate in a deprived urban area in St Helens, Merseyside.

The town depended largely on the coal and glass industries, but following major restructuring in the 1980s lost many jobs which resulted in a further decline in living standards. The area of Thatto Heath chosen for the Rapid Appraisal exercise was representative of the economic and social problems experienced in the town.

The results from this Rapid Appraisal threw up a number of different issues, but also showed similarities with the preoccupations of the Linacre ward community (Table 5.2):

A detailed report on the project was produced (McKenzie *et al.*, 1990) which provided evidence that the area was fragmented physically and socially, despite the fact that family networks were strong and

Table 5.2 Thatto Heath, 1990. Community priorities

Community capacity	
1. General apathy	1.33
2. Absence of a community centre	2.40
3. Large number of single parents	2.87
4. Prejudice against 'outsiders'	3.40
Socio-economic environment	
1. Unemployment	1.60
2. Lack of opportunities	2.53
3. Poverty and deprivation	2.93
4. Poor education	2.93
Physical environment	
1. Lack of security	2.53
2. Little open space	3.20
3. Insufficient housing allocation	4.00
4. Pollution	4.00
5. Rats and rubbish	4.40
6. Dogs	4.67
7. Unsafe roads	5.20
Health, social and environmental services	
1. Services are inadequate	2.47
2. Disabled facilities are poor	2.53
3. No activities for teenagers	3.13
4. No local GP or chemist	3.33
5. Poor information on aids and adaptations	3.53
Disease and disability	
1. Respiratory disease	3.13
2. Excessive smoking and drinking	3.13
3. Chronic illness	3.80
4. Acceptance of ill health as 'normal'	3.93
5. Poor diet	4.13
6. Hard drugs	4.80
7. Lack of parenting skills	5.07
Valuable resources	
1. Supportive family networks	1.87
2. Community spirit	2.00
3. Good informal information network	2.13

supportive. Crime and vandalism were perceived to be high, and unemployment was cited as a key underlying cause of social problems. The prevalent attitude to health was negative and seen as an extension of the feeling of a lack of personal control over many influencing factors.

The report was written to serve as a basis for a community action plan and prominently featured the need to create a general community meeting place. A full list of possible actions was included in the report, and was debated with some vigour by the community. However, the list contained 15 priority issues, which had to be reduced to a manageable size. This involved the community in a further round of commentary, and established a continuous dialogue and the setting of clear action targets.

The main difference between the Thatto Heath and Linacre ward exercises was that in Thatto Heath good longer term relationships with the community could be established. This was partly because some of the team members were already well-known and accepted by the community, partly because the team members were middle managers who were more 'stable' in their post than the senior ranks. The biggest weakness was that few of the middle managers were resource holders, and had to ask permission from their superiors to implement action.

A further exercise attempted to combine the lessons from Linacre and Thatto Heath by drawing together a mix of managers, both from the senior ranks such as a Manager of Nursing Services and the Area Officer for Social Services, with other professionals such as a GP in a large (non-fundholding) practice. This team also included purchasers and providers, based on the belief that needs assessment is the concern of both. The site for this Rapid Appraisal was the Blythe Hill area in London. At the time of writing the research was incomplete, and therefore, no results can be presented. In the same period a group of managers in Northern Ireland worked on the RA methodology with one of the authors of the Linacre exercise (Humphris).

Rapid Appraisal forces managers to adopt a perspective which questions their assumptions and raises doubt about their capacity to determine needs from a purely managerial and professional perspective. If one wants services to be responsive to users, then one has to understand how communities view the world, how they understand the causes of ill health and how health figures in their list of priorities. Managers cannot plan without having some insight into how users interpret their problems, and how they make choices. One way is getting closer to the user and opening up a dialogue, using a systematic and rigorous approach, capable of generating the data required.

The unidentified programme effects of Rapid Appraisal are worth mentioning. Joint working between managers of various organizations was greatly enhanced through the collaboration on the RA exercise. Understanding of each other's professional and organizational background improved and made relationships smoother and more relaxed. This carried over into other meetings and encounters.

Another effect is the resistance from other managers who view the whole enterprise as biased and subjective, or even political, and therefore dismiss both the process and the outcome. It is important to stress the methodological aspects of RA, for example, the use of external facilitators to streamline and focus the process and the various tools for triangulation: multi-agency membership, working in teams rather than as single interviewers, comparing and contrasting data sources, that is, secondary data, observations and interviews. The scientific basis of RA cannot be compromised, and is a necessary requirement for its being a planning tool with broad, genuine and long-term involvement of different organizations and communities.

CONCLUSION

User involvement in health service planning is an important area for development as no established methods exist. Different approaches have been used, but mostly based on community development models without rigorous research protocols. The main challenge is to link systematic research into a community's own perceptions of need with the management process in order to integrate users in the core of policy formulation and strategic decision-making.

The Rapid Appraisal method is still evolving but appears to be capable of presenting a complex picture of priority needs as experienced by a community. However, its main purpose is to formulate action plans which bring together managers and communities, and thus draw (prospective) users into the planning process. The method works well with small, well-defined communities (approximately 10–12 000 inhabitants). Because Rapid Appraisal provides a qualitative perspective on needs it has to be complemented by quantitative methods in order to provide a full picture. Most importantly, commitment to change on the part of managers is an essential precondition for the success of the method and has to be secured from the beginning of the project.

Chapter Six

Evaluation in health services research

INTRODUCTION

Since the introduction of general management in the NHS further major policy changes have made the role of managers in the process of change increasingly important. Paton and Bach (1990) argue that 'the Government has not always been prescriptive about the manner in which policy should be implemented. Instead the onus has been placed on management to fashion policy in the most appropriate way to meet central objectives' (p.4). This is important in the light of the realization that policy, implementation and evaluation are not only overlapping but interacting with each other to produce change (Fazey, 1987, p.2).

In this chapter evaluation is discussed as an integral part of the policy and management processes, and as such has to be planned at the beginning of intended change. It is, therefore, closely linked with the setting of organizational aims and objectives, and framed by the overall goals for the NHS. Managers have, as a result, a key role to play in the shaping of the service, but have an equally important role in the evaluation. Only evaluation which is used to improve the service is worth doing.

The discussion will start with delineating the theoretical basis of evaluation research, and outlines the conceptual framework. The design of evaluation studies and methodological options will be reviewed, and two case studies are detailed. The first case deals with the organizational impact of the use of minimally invasive therapies; the second case evaluates the quality of life of people discharged from a large mental institution to community settings.

EVALUATION RESEARCH

Evaluation is recognized as important, yet there is no agreed definition as to what it is and what it should do. Daly and McDonald (1992) point out that there are considerable uncertainties with regard to the state of knowledge about effectiveness in health care and how to evaluate effectiveness. This is not merely a technical problem of method, but the social aspects of practice and change in practice can no longer be ignored.

Fazey (1987) provides a thought-provoking discussion of this issue, but opts for the broad definition by Rossi which sees evaluation as 'the application of social science knowledge and research methods to the assessment of social programmes'. In choosing this definition the present discussion excludes other forms of evaluation such as clinical procedures, or specific methods such as cost-effectiveness analysis. Evaluating health services in this more technical way has been described by St Leger *et al.*, (1992) when they define health service evaluation as 'the critical assessment, on as objective a basis as possible, of the degree to which entire services or their component parts (e.g. diagnostic tests, caring procedures) fulfil stated goals' (p.1).

Evaluation as discussed in this chapter draws on the social sciences, and focuses on organizational and socio-cultural issues relating to health. To put it in concrete terms, it addresses questions such as whether the implementation of policy, for example discharging people from long-stay institutions to the community, leads to an improvement of health service practice and quality of life of users and providers of that service. The goals of change will be critically reviewed within the evaluation, and are not taken as given. Fazey (1987) points out that defining goals is problematic because one can distinguish operative goals from official goals. Different groups within an organization may have different goals, not only from each other, but also from the organization as a whole. Understanding goal 'dissonance' is important at the start of an evaluation, in order to formulate the various standards operated by different interest groups. Furthermore, even if shared goals can be established the interpretation and implementation of these goals can vary.

These considerations are important as they directly relate to the aim of evaluation. Lyons Morris *et al.* (1987) argue that an evaluation cannot be free from political considerations, and therefore one has to know the motivations and idiosyncrasies of the people for whom the evaluation is intended. Different users will want the evaluation to support their own particular point of view, and the evaluation researcher has to be aware of these differences in order to design the research in a balanced manner.

Bulmer (1986) warns that the policy-making process itself is one of conflictual negotiation between groups. Social science research is capable of making a contribution through analysis of objectives, processes and outcomes of policy initiatives.

Illsley (1980) argues that in essence the scientific aims of evaluators in field settings are no different from those of laboratory scientists or exponents of randomized controlled trials. He states that they are similarly concerned with proof, evidence, reliability, validity and so on, but they have to adapt to imposed conditions, which are often determined by policy or strategy. He continues that evaluation then becomes a methodology which aims to produce best approximations to the otherwise unknowable relationships between cause and effect, or between input and output. Furthermore, the data collection methods are varied – historical evidence, documents, records, interviews, survey and so on (p.117).

From the researcher's perspective, two broad approaches can be selected. These are described by Marsden and Oakley (1991) as follows: first, the instrumental/technocratic approach. This represents the dominant paradigm in the field of evaluation studies. It perceives the management task as the development of rationally designed and operational tools for the realization of objectives. Evaluation serves to increase managerial control through the systematic coordination of social action, and tends to be based on a systems approach. Fazey (1987) quotes Allison, who defines the systems management model as one which captures the organizational assumptions of the mainstream, rationalist tradition of policy analysis, and its point of departure is the assumption of value-maximizing behaviour. This approach ignores the political nature of evaluation, as it considers itself value-free and relying on neutral methods.

The second approach is called interpretative and places subjectivity at the centre of human experience. This approach examines the latent functions of evaluations in reinforcing certain forms of social control. It concerns itself with uncovering the political processes involved in evaluations. Evaluations are important critical moments in institutional life, and afford the opportunity to reappraise current practice, and re-formulate objectives, both at the level of policy and implementation. As such this type of evaluation creates openings for other considerations such as participation, capacity building, empowerment, and provides a basis for what Marsden and Oakley call a 'practical' evaluation methodology, directed towards change and improvement.

Taking the perspective of the user of evaluation research, most commonly decision-makers, Bulmer (1986) distinguishes two purposes that evaluation serves in aiding them to reach conclusions about policies: first, formative evaluation which produces information that is fed back during the implementation of policy in order to help improve it. Second, summative evaluation which is carried out once a policy has been implemented, to assess the overall effectiveness of the policy at the end of the implementation process.

Whilst the nature of evaluation research remains an issue for debate, and often is linked to moral and political value judgements, the above discussion has pointed out various perspectives on the role and function of policy evaluation research. The social science approach taken in this book is directed towards engagement, that is, being grounded in the real world where policy makers and managers have to make choices. But underlying these choices, questions have to be answered about the motives behind interventions, about purpose and about process. Evaluation helps to make choices, and St Leger *et al.* (1992) state this in precise terms for senior health service managers who have to:

1. determine clearly what their alternatives are;
2. estimate the likely consequences stemming from each alternative and its chances of occurrence;
3. define clearly what their preferences are;
4. take the alternative which maximizes the expected value (p.182).

Taken within the context of interpretative evaluation, health service managers have to be able to be accountable for their choices, not only 'upwards' – ultimately to the Government – but also 'downwards' to the staff who provide the service directly, and to the (potential) users. Thus, the process of choice itself is one of shared control in setting goals, definitions and expected outcomes. The design of evaluation research, and selected methods, need to be based upon this understanding.

Steps in evaluation research

The aim of the evaluation is the first issue that has to be clarified. This sounds easier than it is, and often has to be negotiated, not only between the evaluator and those who commission the study, but often also between different 'stakeholders' in the commissioning group. It regularly happens that the various aims of the evaluation only emerge during the course of the study demonstrating the distinction between operative and formal goals.

A key element of the assessment of social programmes is to establish the aims of the social/health programme itself. In the same way as the aims of the evaluation can vary, so can the definition of aims of a programme have numerous interpretations and operational guises. Yet, each evaluation has to assess whether an organization or programme achieves the goals that it has set, whether consensus about goals exists or not. If there are multiple non-consensual goals, all have to be discovered and defined in order to draw the baseline for the research.

Once aims and objectives are described the four main elements that have to be evaluated are input, process, outcomes and impact. Input evaluation is, in theory, the most straightforward and relies on accurate information about resources and skills. In the NHS the data sources can be activity data, Korner data sets, patient information systems, medical audit, skill mix data, etc (St Leger *et al.*, 1992).

Process evaluation attempts to capture a 'still frame' of the dynamics and characteristics of an operational, ongoing service programme. It entails the description of the organizational structure, its culture and the relationships within and between relevant groups. It also examines the relationship of the organization with the world around it, for example, the health service has to increasingly look at its relationship with other organizations, user groups and individual users.

Outcome evaluation tries to determine if a programme or project has met its own objectives, and therefore documents change over time, describes specific 'products', for example, behavioural change from a health promotion activity, and relates outcomes to the stated objectives.

Impact evaluation attempts to assess the longer term and generalized results of programme operations. This is the most difficult, and often avoided, aspect of evaluation research. If done properly, it should include a before and after design, that is, to study people before and after a specific intervention, and then follow them up over a long period of time. It is capable of identifying unanticipated effects, and examining those within context. For example, a succesful hip replacement means that some one can walk again, but also has to spend money on buying normal footwear or trousers. Thus, the impact is an unanticipated financial outlay.

Many evaluation studies are not sufficiently long in duration to fully assess impact, but if so, move into the arena of future scenario development. Bezold (1991) puts two assumptions forward: first, the future is uncertain, which means that the forecasts about health and health care are equally uncertain. At the same time, key trends and alternative futures can be mapped in order to get a handle on the future, and possible impacts of health policy and management. Second, managers choose and create major aspects of the future by what they do or fail to do. Thus, large aspects of the future are controllable; for example, the extension of minimally invasive therapies will commit resources and direct professional skills, thereby determining the shape of clinical practice and organizational arrangements.

For a study to incorporate all four levels of evaluation a complex design has to be constructed capable of answering questions at the different levels. An elegant example is provided by Smith and Cantley (1985) who designed an evaluation of a psycho-geriatric day hospital. They examined the various ways in which participants assessed the performance of the unit and identified six major categories. These categories were then used as the basis for an evaluation of the unit, by collecting, organizing and analysing the data following these six categories. This meant that they remained close to the way participants had defined these terms and assessed organizational performance against this framework. This approach allowed them to distinguish between different objectives pursued by the various (groups of) participants, and to place ideas and actions within a broader context.

The techniques involved in evaluation research depend on the purpose: when addressing input a descriptive method can be employed providing an accurate picture of resources, using a range of secondary data sources, alongside newly collected survey and interview material. Process evaluation is most commonly done by analysing documents which are tracing developments over time, for example reports, minutes of meetings, by interview (mostly ethnographic) and (participant) observation. This will release comparative material capable of relating significant variables to each other and assessing their impact on the functioning of the programme under study.

Studying outcome and impact can be done through experimental design, or a before and after design using standardized instruments. Variations on these methods include using the study group as its own control. Basically explanatory information is collected answering the question of why a particular programme works, thus attempting to establish a level of causality or formulating a set of preconditions and key variables for success. At its most sophisticated level it can be used to test theory or build models.

Fazey (1987) constructs a matrix which includes the above mentioned dimensions, and adds four targets for evaluative research. She argues that evaluation can be targeted at the individual, the programme, the service system of which the programme is part, or society as a whole. The process, outcome and impact are different for each target area, and can contradict each other. This complexity has to be understood if the results of an evaluation are to be implemented.

Lyons Morris *et al.* (1987) emphasize the importance of communicating evaluation findings in such a way as to ensure optimal action. Given the understanding of evaluation as crucial in the improvement of practice, and the health management context which requires services to be explicit about its costs and benefits, acting upon findings has to be ensured. However, similar difficulties arise as with the setting of objectives. For example, different users want different types of information, even to answer the same question. The evaluation has to be sufficiently flexible to give these different answers.

The situation where people cannot see the benefit of an evaluation is not uncommon, and evaluation researchers have to clarify what the evaluation information can achieve. On the other hand, managers can expect the evaluation to confirm their opinion, and the presentation of alternative truths is the main evaluation task. Furthermore, information needs can change during the evaluation, as new insights are emerging which alter the original conception of the study. Lyons Morris *et al.* (1987) argue that if one wants managers to listen to and act upon the evaluation findings, attention has to be paid to what exactly they want to know; that is, what are the various objectives for the evaluation?

In conclusion, evaluation research is aimed at assessing social programmes in order to aid decision-making. The definition of evaluation research is not only the prerogative of managers and researchers, but has to include a level of accountability upwards and downwards in order to widen control and empowerment for change. Therefore, evaluation cannot be seen as a pure technical exercise, but primarily as a social one, involving choices and alternatives. Bulmer (1986) adds that social scientists as evaluators offer both methodological know-how and theoretical understanding. This implies a claim to independent knowledge, and as such analysis and action remain distinct. In order to fulfil this promise of insightful knowledge in the policy process, evaluation research has to adhere to scientific standards, and to be capable of embracing the full range of methods, emphasizing their interpretative power.

CASE 1   THE ORGANIZATIONAL IMPACT OF MINIMALLY INVASIVE THERAPY

The background

Minimally invasive therapy (MIT) is an area of medical treatment that causes substantially reduced trauma to the person undergoing it. In part it is made up of changing techniques, but it also depends in most cases on new and advanced technologies, especially endoscopes and imaging devices (Banta, 1991). The development of MIT in developed countries has accelerated in the last decade, and in the UK the advances are keeping pace with the rest of Europe. At the same time, considered against the structural and strategic changes in the NHS, the further development of MIT is becoming more unpredictable (Ong, 1993).

Innovations in medical practice have to be understood within the complex context of the NHS and the national economy at large. At the same time, processes within the medical profession and the health service institutions influence the development and diffusion of new approaches such as MIT. On the one hand, innovations are communicated through the social system through 'product champions' and adapters (Stocking, 1984); on the other hand, older paradigms are replaced by new incompatible ones, which affect the culture and organization of the scientific community (Kuhn, 1970) and society at large. Thus, innovations have an organizational impact beyond the boundaries of the medical scientific community, and it is this impact which is the subject of the evaluation study.

The organizational study

The study of the organizational impact of MIT was part of a larger EC-funded project examining the processes of diffusion and barriers to diffusion of MIT in five European countries. The aim of the organizational study was to evaluate the impact of the introduction of MIT on the different groups working within and using the services of the organization. The objectives of the study were to analyse the organizational processes taking place with the introduction of new technology, to describe the expected and intended outcomes and to assess the impact on users' perceptions of care, both within the institutional and community settings.

Organizations can be defined as social entities that have a purpose and a boundary, so that some participants are considered inside while others are considered outside, and this patterns activities of particpants into a recognizable structure (Daft, 1989). Sociologists have been particularly interested in understanding organizations within their contextual setting of a wider societal and institutional framework (Butler, 1991). Pettigrew (1990) has argued that in order to understand the continuity and change in organizations the research approach should be contextual and processual in character. This includes both multilevel and processual analysis, emphasizing the importance of interconnectedness between the levels of analysis, of historical understanding and of the link between context and action. Anthropologists focus on the interpretative frameworks of the actors involved in the processes of change. Here, the emphasis is placed on unfolding change and how different perspectives are required at different times in the process (Isabella, 1990). An evaluation of an organization subject to change through the introduction of new technologies can best be studied by applying an evaluative model based on the above two theoretical approaches. This model mirrors many of the concerns of the interpretative evaluation discussed earlier, and the structure outlined by Fazey (1987).

In consequence, the research design is a dynamic one, aimed at understanding the complexity of the various processes taking place at the different levels. At the same time, the study, like many management projects, was very time limited and had to take a multilayered still frame, rather than a horizontal picture.

The research design

The process–outcome–impact framework was followed in the study of the selected organization, which was the National Medical Laser Centre in London. This Centre received Special Medical Development funding from the Government between 1986 and 1992 in order to develop lasers for clinical practice. The Centre operates as a specialist facility, taking referrals from outside its own district. The Centre carries out clinical and experimental work, and at the end of the SMD funding the host District has to pay for the routine clinical laser service.

For the specific study only the laser treatments for people with advanced cancer of the oesophagus were evaluated. The reasons for selecting this particular client group were two-fold: first, a randomized controlled trial carried out by the Centre team was under way, including quality of life measures of people suffering from cancer of the oesophagus; second, this client group represented a large proportion of the cancer-related work in the Centre.

The design was built around sequential steps, with firstly, process being studied in the following ways:

- The objectives of the new technology (laser therapy for people with oesophageal cancer) had to be described by the various actors: medical staff, nurses, managers, users, referrers and carers.
- The target population had to be identified, and the criteria for inclusion/exclusion defined. Decision-making structures based on these criteria had to be analysed.
- A description of the services delivered within the organization had to be furnished.
- A description of the systems of evaluation, quality assurance and medical audit had to be given, and their modes of operation.
- An analysis of the relationships and patterns of interaction within the organization and with those outside had to be made.

Secondly, outcome had to be examined through:

- understanding definitions of success, i.e. whether a programme of MIT (in this case laser therapy) met its own objectives as defined in clinical and managerial terms;
- how referring agents are defining success;
- how users and carers define success, especially in relation to quality of life, or in comparison to alternative or more invasive procedures.

Thirdly, impact had to be assessed through:

- estimating the longer term effects on the internal organization, specifically in relation to clinical practice, modalities of nursing and other supportive care during and after the therapy;

- estimating the effects of laser therapy on community services and informal care in the home.

The Centre study was structured as a case study, utilizing various methodological devices, including the collection of secondary data, such as service uptake, research reports, medical audit data. Primary data collection was done through non-participant observation in the clinic and on the ward, and semi-structured interviews of key personnel. Furthermore, an opportunistic sample of users was interviewed either immediately before or after treatment (that is, whilst still in hospital). A small sample of referrers was interviewed by telephone as their geographical spread was nationwide.

The themes for the interviews followed the format of process–outcome–impact, which meant that the discussion was structured to address the issues within each stage. The ethnographic interview method was used, with notes taken rather than tape-recording. The material emerging from the interviews was triangulated, to make comparisons both between groups and within groups.

Selected findings

Using an interpretative evaluation on an organization delivers a certain type of findings. They are predominantly focused on dynamics of the organization, relationships and perceptions, and as such can provide insight into how change in one part of the organization affects other parts. This is precisely what happened in the Laser Centre study.

The introduction of laser technology was driven by the medical profession, whose objectives were two-fold: first, service-oriented, because they were confronted with the problem of an incurable and distressing type of cancer, namely oesophageal cancer. They wanted to alleviate patients' suffering and searched for treatments which at least could palliate the most distressing symptoms, mainly the inability to swallow. Second, this search fuelled the research objective which was to further develop and improve therapies, and compare with alternatives in order to establish the most effective and cost-effective combination of treatments.

The nursing profession focused on the quality of life issues, and the provision of holistic nursing care. They emphasized the need to operate a 'seamless' service between hospital and community, and prioritized good communication. This also included communication with the patients, which at times could be difficult because they were referred from other hospitals without necessarily knowing the nature of their disease. Palliative laser therapy tends to require only a couple of days in hospital, and is administered on an intermittent basis. This meant that nurses did have limited opportunity to get to know the 'whole person'. Thus, the treatment itself required a re-orientation of nursing objectives and practice, with nurses not necessarily sharing the research aims.

For managers laser treatments meant reducing in-patient stay, and as a result, changing planning and organizational procedures. Important logistical issues such as transport and after-care had to be addressed in order to benefit fully from the opportunities afforded by reduced bed occupancy. However, not all back-up systems could be fully developed or controlled, and the treatment itself had a margin of unpredictability, thus requiring managers to plan more flexibly. The funding of the Centre created a separate set of issues: Districts were willing to buy routine laser treatments, but did not pay for experimental work. Within the new contract culture research and development remained a grey area, and caused much concern among managers and clinicians.

The main objective for the users was to be relieved from the symptoms of disease. However, the palliative nature of the treatment was not fully understood by everyone, resulting in a lack of clarity about expectations. Reduced hospital stay was generally seen as positive, but users emphasized the importance of back-up services such as transport and home care. The need for support and advice after discharge was underlined, and outreach from the hospital was seen as most appropriate.

The referring clinicians considered the laser treatment as a necessary episode in the process of care, and emphasized that they wanted to retain control over the management of individual patients' treatment regimens.

In terms of outcome, the medical profession used the findings from their RCT as a yardstick. This RCT measured survival and quality of life, with swallowing as the main indicator. For nurses, outcome was primarily quality of life. The extension of life was a difficult issue as the boundaries between palliative care and terminal care could become blurred, and nurses considered being free of pain and discomfort the key outcome measures. These were outcomes expressed by users themselves; however, length of life was frequently mentioned as of equal importance. Managers intended to use a cost-benefit analysis to determine outcomes but because of the unpredictable nature of the treatment and as yet insufficient evidence, were unable to come up with unambiguous yardsticks. Instead, throughput and control of resources were proxy outcome measures, awaiting the results of medical audit, RCT data and the results of the cost-effectiveness study (Sculpher and Buxton, 1991).

Assessing the impact of laser treatment for people with cancer of the oesophagus will remain difficult while their lifespan is limited to an average of 6–12 months. At the same time, there are indications that the provision of a seamless service is a priority if the quality of life is to be enhanced. In terms of the treatment itself, it is to be expected that lasers will increasingly be used in the future, because of the positive impact on the financing of palliative care through short treatment and inpatient care. However, hard evidence from cost-effectivness research is, as yet, not available. Its acceptability to users and referrers points towards increased future use.

By employing a process–outcome–impact framework for the interpretative evaluation the different objectives, perceptions and indicators for success could be uncovered. Further exploration of relationships and cost-effectiveness issues would have been able to give the impact analysis a firmer conceptual and empirical basis, but at present the study allows a broad framework for analysis. The managerial issues of understanding the nature and scope of new technologies and their impact on other parts of the service are important for their decision-making about resources, skill mix, communications with other providers and developing new service approaches. In this sense, the research has taken on the character of a formative evaluation whereby issues are highlighted in ways not previously recognized, and thereby informing the decision-making process.

The evaluation study opens up avenues of thinking beyond the costs of introducing a new technology into changing objectives, clinical and nursing practice and the implications for formal and informal care in the community. This means that questions can be posed about how well the procedure works in practice, whether it meets the criteria of human care and whether the benefits are equally distributed (Daly and McDonald, 1992).Only when the totality of the experience of treatment is addressed can improvements in service make a fundamental impact on people's quality of life.

CASE 2   THE QUALITY OF LIFE OF PEOPLE DISCHARGED FROM LONG-STAY INSTITUTIONS

The background

The policy of de-institutionalization of mental health care has been implemented with differences in pace and scope because the central policy has been interpreted and implemented with considerable local variation (Tomlinson, 1991). The reduction of places in long-stay institutions has been the subject of national and local debate, and has been scrutinized by a variety of agencies, including the Audit Commission (1986), the National Schizophrenia Fellowship (1985) and MIND (1989–90). There has been considerable criticism of the policies and practices aimed at responding to the needs of people discharged into the community, most notably highlighted in the Griffiths report on

Community Care (1988) which formed the basis for the White Paper *Caring for People* (DoH, 1989a). An issue that has received most attention in the last few years has been the link between mental health and homelessness (Williams and Allen, 1989).

On the other hand, positive assessments have documented relative successes (PSSRU, 1987) and theoretical work advancing the principles underlying community services has made a substantive contribution to philosophical, social policy and management thinking.

Despite the plethora of research and policy documents, relatively little work has been carried out into the quality of life of people in provisions other than long-stay institutions. Research has taken place on specific projects (Kay and Legg, 1986; Harpurhey Resettlement Project, 1987; Clifford and Holloway, 1989), or lessons can be learned from research in comparative fields (O'Brien and Tyne, 1981; Baldwin *et al.*, 1990). In particular, the work on quality of life is important, and can draw on general theoretical literature (Williams, 1985 and 1987). Holmes (1989) argues that developing objective measures are problematic and states that an individual's quality of life cannot be abstracted from his/her social context and assessed in isolation. This is an important considera-tion when studying people discharged from long-stay institutions who have to (re)build a social context for themselves.

Furthermore, the population leaving long-stay institutions is unique in that their needs are qualitatively different from other people with mental health problems, mainly related to the impact of institutionalization on their personality and social relations. Although inappropriate admissions which become long-stay are intended to be a thing of the past, populations with chronic and complex mental health problems will pose continuing challenges. Therefore, it is not only important to understand the needs and quality of life of those people leaving long-stay institutions, but also what we can learn from their experiences for other client groups with similar difficulties.

The study

Hilltop Health Authority has been operating a programme of rehabilita-tion, discharge and community care at its large long-stay institution with the aim of reducing the patient population to around 200 people. The aim of the programme was to provide individuals with suitable accommoda-tion which would allow them to contribute whatever they were capable of, providing an opportunity for personal development towards greater personal responsibility and independence, or alternatively, continued supervision on a much less formal basis than provided by long-term hospital care (Hilltop HA report on rehabilitation).

With the introduction of the National Health Service and Community Care Act 1990 individual Health Authorities and relevant Social Services Departments will agree the exact form of local care programming for people with mental health problems (DoH, 1990, p.80). This means that service levels have to be defined more precisely, and care plans with an indefinite time limit and unspecified service input cannot be sustained. Therefore, a clear assessment of needs has to be made at both an individual and client group level, an analysis of available skills and resources has to be carried out and statements about outcomes in terms of quality of life have to be developed.

Hilltop Health Authority wanted to establish what levels of support existed for people with long-term mental health problems who were living in the community in order to assess the resources needed to implement care management. Therefore, a study defining quality of life, and analysing the level of co-ordination and support needed to achieve good quality of life, was deemed necessary in order to provide guidance for the distribution of resources within a community setting. In order to generate quality of life concepts a study evaluating the quality of life of people currently living in the community (and who were previously residents in the long-stay institution) was commissioned, and executed by the Centre for Health Planning and Management.

The overall aims of the study were:

1. to define the elements which constitute quality of life, both for client groups and individuals;
2. to assess whether and, if so, how quality can be incorporated in objective setting for service providers and for individual clients;
3. to asess whether and, if so, how the provision of rehabilitation services contributes to individuals' quality of life;
4. to assess whether quality of life can be used as an outcome measure.

The research design

The evaluation study was used in order to develop understanding of the experience of living in community settings by assessing people's quality of life. Because of the lack of available tools to assess the quality of life of this particular client group no standards could be used to evaluate against. Unusually, therefore, this evaluation approach was used to formulate dimensions of the concept of quality of life and, in a way, aimed to arrive at a post hoc definition.

The concept of quality of life was to be studied in two ways: first, to assess the quality of life of the particular client group as a whole, i.e. people who have been institutionalized for a number of years; second, to assess the quality of life of individual clients.

The interpretative evaluation was designed as follows:

1. to carry out a restrospective study of eight clients who have been resettled in the community, and who represent the four major settings available in Hilltop;
2. a three month longitudinal study of eight clients discharged to Brookfield hostel in 1989 (to start one month before discharge);
3. a study of a sample of service providers (doctors, nurses, social workers, occupational therapists, rehabilitation managers, hostel and home managers) matched with the clients in 1 and 2 above;
4. a study of relatives and friends of the clients in 1 and 2 above.

The sample

Hilltop Health Authority has used four different types of community settings for placing people discharged from their long-stay institution, namely hostels and group homes (28), elderly people homes (16), private homes (13) and people that have been directly discharged into their own independent living accommodation (30). Two people were randomly selected from each subgroup for interview. They were approached by their Community Psychiatric Nurse or social worker to ask their co-operation with the study. When they had given consent the researcher made an appointment to interview them at a mutually convenient time.

For each client the key worker was interviewed, which could, for example, be a social worker, CPN or a hostel manager. One or two significant others were selected by each client, and approached for interview by the researcher. They included parents, brothers or sisters and a vicar.

One group home with eight people, Brookfield hostel, was selected to be studied in its totality, from inception to two months after opening. All inhabitants were interviewed before leaving hospital, and at least twice after moving into the hostel. All members of staff were interviewed on a formal or informal basis during these three months.

The key local policy makers were interviewed, including the Specialty Managers for rehabilitation services, Director of Nursing, Specialty Director/consultant psychiatrist and Team Manager (CPNs).

Methods of data collection

Two strategies were formulated, one for the random sample of eight clients living in three different community settings, the other for the group of clients living in Brookfield. This can be represented as in Figure 6.1.

	subgroup 1	subgroup 2 Brookfield
Secondary data (policy and strategy documents, assessments)	yes	yes
Non-participant observation	no	yes
Ethnographic interview of self	yes	yes
Ethnographic interview of key worker	yes	yes
Ethnographic interview of significant others	yes	yes

Figure 6.1 Data collection methods

The study of Brookfield was carried out using a pluralistic case study approach (Smith and Cantley, 1985). Figure 6.1 shows the different methods employed, which constituted a mixture of timetabled and opportunistic research. Thus, a series of pre-arranged interviews were carried out, the first one being a group interview when the clients were still in hospital, and being prepared for discharge. The second interview was done with individuals within a fortnight of having moved to the new unit, while subsequent interviews were opportunistic, that is, taking place during informal visits to the hostel. The interviews were thematic and chronologically ordered. The themes covered included decision-making about the future, preparation for discharge, choices on new living environment, problems, activities and social contacts, feelings about life in the community, indicators used for determining one's quality of life. All interviews took the form of a conversation and the pre-arranged interviews were tape-recorded with the client's consent, and transcripts were given to the interviewee for approval. Informal discussions were noted down after the visit.

During the visits informal discussions took place with members of staff, while more formal interviews were also organized, which again were thematic. They covered assessment, preparation, choice for clients, problems, levels of support, activities and social contacts, communications with other service providers, community care policies locally and nationally, indicators for quality of life. These interviews were tape-recorded and transcribed for approval from the respondent.

Non-participant observation took place during the formal and informal visits, and notes were taken afterwards. These formed the background against which the operational policy of the hostel could be tested. It also provided the context for assessing the relationships between residents, and between staff and residents, and could form the frame of reference against which to evaluate quality of life statements.

The main method for studying the sample of people living in EPHs, other hostels or private homes and in independent living accommodation was through in-depth interviews. Each client was interviewed once, using the same thematic format as for the group discussed above. The interviews were tape-recorded and transcripts were sent back for approval.

The sample of significant others was interviewed in two ways: either personally (some were tape-recorded, while others only wanted notes to be taken) or through a telephone conversation. The themes addressed in these interviews were involvement in decision-making and preparation for discharge, problems encountered by client, support provided for client and self, assessment of client's activities and social contacts, opinion on the national and local policies for community care and indicators of the client's quality of life.

The secondary data was collected to gain insight in evolving perceptions over time, and to follow through the key decision-making stages. The assessments were used to examine the criteria for discharge, so that comparisons could be made between professional and client (relatives) assessment of need and preference.

Fundamentally, the interview data formed the backbone of the study, whilst the secondary and observational material was used in a comparative manner (triangulation, which is to be discussed in the chapter on multimethod research). The main method of analysis was the grounded theory approach (Glaser and Strauss, 1967) which represented a distinct perspective on the analysis of qualitative data for the discovery and understanding of social processes. This approach built up theoretical understanding from an in-depth analysis of 'rich' data through classification, the identification of properties, the making of conceptual linkages and relationships to building concepts. The experiential material collected in this study lent itself to this methodological approach, and was consistent with the research aim of using an evaluative approach to understand which elements were indicative for quality of life.

Main findings

The report for Hilltop Health Authority was written in an ethnographic style, addressing the aims of the study. The thematically organized findings can be summarized as follows: the process of discharge and settling people into a new living environment is a key indicator of how services contribute to the individual's quality of life. In anthropological theory, the concept of status passage helps to explain the complex changes in role and self-perception that individuals go through when major transitions take place in their life (Glaser and Strauss, 1967). For people who have previously lived in institutions, the status passage to living in the community is multifaceted: they make the transition from inmate to citizen, which involves new expectations and obligations, understanding the prevalent social and cultural codes, participating in community-based social life and taking on different responsibilities.

The study demonstrated that the areas most affected by this transition were the daily routine of caring for oneself, work and comparable activities, and relationships with others. In terms of quality of life people had to be given the opportunity to develop self-care skills as a basic requirement for maintenance within a community setting. A minority appeared to be succesful in obtaining work, or in participating in meaningful activities such as church work. Reliance on the individual's personal strength was insufficient, and an explicit advocacy role had to be undertaken by service providers in order to create opportunities open to other members of society. To plan and monitor people's needs in taking opportunities contributed to their quality of life.

Maintenance of individuals' health and well-being has been shown to depend on the existence of social relationships. Goldberg and Hillier (1979) argued that social isolation is a clear indicator of mental health problems. Thus, quality of life can be gauged by the level and nature of social contacts.

Social contacts of the study population appeared to be largely confined to historical relationships carried over from the hospital period, or new contacts were made within a community-based group living situation. New contacts outside those two contexts were established by only a handful of people. Creating one's own social environment 'from scratch' after a prolonged period outside normal society is a tall order, especially if people have been de-skilled in social intercourse. Planned support in creating new networks and access to community resources was necessary to improve this quality of life dimension.

One of the central arguments for advocating de-institutionalization has been to increase an individual's locus of control. Goffman (1961) and others have convincingly demonstrated that institutional life diminishes people's capacity to determine their own destiny. The move to the community is intended to remedy this and bring it in line with the normal citizen. This immediately poses a theoretical problem, as the locus of control differs for different social groups and individuals within those groups, depending on socio-economic status, gender, race, domestic responsibilities, duties at work.

The aspects most discussed in the literature are tangible ones such as choice of living environment, control over financial resources or personal time. The users in this study mentioned these issues as important, while two people who were living by themselves addressed the more fundamental question of determining one's own destiny. They explained the type of choices they had made about the shape of their life, and the reasons for not adhering to cultural stereotypes, for example, pursuing a career.

The most important dimension of quality of life appeared to be the notion of freedom. Most clients understood this freedom also to entail responsibility, because it was determined within the boundaries of social obligations and cultural norms. But mostly, freedom was defined as a relative concept, namely in comparison with institutional life. It was interesting to note that people did not redefine their frame of reference by comparing their new situation with the dominant culture or a particular social grouping. Instead, they used a historical frame of reference, i.e. the hospital situation, and subsequently judged that their quality of life had improved because of greater freedom and control.

In contrast, relatives and friends were embedded in the framework of the dominant culture and its values. They used more absolute indicators of quality of life, and placed great value on individuality and personal achievement. This was exemplified in their aspirations that their relative would find a partner, a job and participate in a range of social activities.

Despite relatives and friends having different aspirations for them, the majority of people who left hospital felt that they were in the right place, considering their own skills and mental state. Holmes (1989) argues that quality of life should fulfil two fundamental needs:

1. to avoid and/or adjust to painful experiences;
2. to develop and sustain life satisfaction by increasing competency, skills and mastery over the environment.

The people interviewed illustrated this argument by stating the boundaries to their choices, and as such determined the degree of quality of life they could cope with and accept. At the same time, quality of life is not a given and static situation. The biggest challenge to service providers lies in their ability to respond to evolving needs.

Implications for management

Quality of life of people discharged to community settings is not a unitary concept. Rather, it is determined by a person's past and present social context. The definition operates at two levels: first, in terms of fundamental human values; second, as a dynamic concept that has to be connected to an individual's own perceptions and expectations. By implication, service provision has to be able to adapt. Needs have to be assessed in a process of regular re-examination with the client in order to design flexible packages of care.

In parallel, targets have to be set with the client about the levels of quality of life he or she hopes to achieve, which determines the amount and nature of professional input required. This can provide a framework for collaboration and a division of labour between different agencies, and between the client and those agencies. The study did not provide conclusive estimations of the contribution of rehabilitation services to the client's quality of life. However, research on the use of a problem-oriented method of quality assurance has made the link between therapeutic input and outcome in individuals (McDonald and Blizard, 1988). If targets are set the contribution of the formal and informal agencies can be defined and co-ordinated in order to achieve defined quality of life outcomes.

The study showed, in common with other similar studies (for example on the needs of carers, Twigg *et al.*, 1990), that a client's social network has different needs. Meeting those needs can have a positive effect on the client's quality of life. When families and friends know they can have access to professional support in their task of helping the client, they are often willing to be integrated in the caring network, as proposed in the *Caring for People* document.

The type of evaluation that was asked for by the commissioning managers straddled the boundaries of summative and formative evaluation. The emphasis on the quality of life meant that this was seen as the main indicator to determine the success of the local approach to de-institutionalization. At the same time, the concept of quality had to be defined in the course of the study, and as such the evaluation was formative, allowing new interpretations to inform ongoing policy and practice.

Because of this hybrid project brief certain key questions could not be fully answered. Managers' objectives encompassed the implementation of national policy and the desire to develop a value-led mental health service aimed at extended people's capacity.

CONCLUSION

Evaluation research is inherently political, as it is directly linked with the objectives of a social programme, and with more general managerial aims and objectives. This chapter has discussed the different purposes evaluation serves: it is primarily a management tool, which assists in understanding whether objectives are achieved. At the same time it represents a critical moment in the life of an organization as it is also capable of questioning objectives, either organizational or those of the evaluation itself. It can be argued that real evaluation has to be used to reformulate policy and implementation, if deemed necessary, rather than justify current decision-making and operations.

Evaluation research helps managers to make choices. The two case studies demonstrated different aspects of choice. The first one uncovered the complex interplay of perceptions of different groups within an organization, and the ripple effect of a change in medical practice on policy and implementation. The evaluation enabled managers to gain an overview of this complexity and to make choices about the future investments, direction and shape of the service.

The second case used evaluation to sharpen understanding about a key concept in judging the success of a policy. The implicit assumption of transferring people from mental institutions to community settings is that it improves their quality of life. However, the definition of this concept was far from clear, and the evaluation study allowed users' own definitions of quality to influence conceptual thinking of policy makers and managers. This indirectly addressed the question of control in evaluation, and the problem that Marsden and Oakley (1991) raised about empowerment.

The cases illustrated that within the overall evaluation approach, and the structure for examining process, outcome and impact, the research design has to be sufficiently flexible to address the specific evaluation question. The first case focused more strictly on evaluation, while the second case used evaluation to further develop concepts. Despite the difference in emphasis, the common elements in both cases have been the interpretative nature of the evaluation method, and a design that is capable of extracting precisely the necessary subjective material, alongside the more quantitative comparative data. Managers will have to employ this type of approach if evaluation research is to provide answers to their questions about policy and implementation.

Chapter Seven

Multimethod research

INTRODUCTION

The previous chapters have dealt with the main social science research methods, but implicitly have not just focused on one method at a time. For example, when carrying out a Rapid Appraisal, the dominant approach is qualitative interviewing, but the collection and re-analysis of secondary data is an important part of the total research process. This chapter will deal explicitly with the design of research projects utilizing more than one method at a time, and discuss the reasons for choosing multimethod research.

Health service managers are dealing with increasingly complex issues, and because of this complexity research intended to clarify issues and provide solutions cannot rely on one 'all-singing, all-dancing' method. When examining specific case studies such as the assessment of need, it rapidly becomes clear that the concept of need is multifaceted, and requires to be studied from different vantage points. The health service perspective on need relies on an analysis of service utilization data and professional assessments, whilst the user perspective emphasizes the impact of disease on the totality of living. Each perspective demands a different methodology, both elucidating 'need'.

In this chapter the principles of multimethod research will be discussed, and two case studies illustrate this approach. Firstly, the assessment of need of the over–75 population in general practice; secondly, a needs and quality of life study on people with physical disabilities in a small town. In multimethod research design issues are most important, and this chapter elaborates more on research decision-making than on the results of study.

PRINCIPLES OF MULTIMETHOD RESEARCH

Each research methodology has its particular strengths, but also its weaknesses. For example, the controlled experiment can test hypotheses and demonstrate causal relationships between variables, but precisely because of the controlled circumstances it is difficult to estimate whether the responses of the experimental subjects occur in the same way under natural conditions. The realization that each method has specific weaknesses has given rise to the multimethod approach.

Brewer and Hunter (1989) argue that although individual methods may be flawed, fortunately the flaws in each are not identical. They see the fundamental strategy of the multimethod approach as being 'to attack a research problem with an arsenal of methods that have non-overlapping weaknesses in addition to their complementary strengths' (p.17). This also results in the generation of multiple data sets about the same research problem, each set being collected with a different type of method. Thus, they argue that the main advantage of the multimethod approach is its ability to deliver a diversity in data, and therefore, the opportunity for detailed comparison (p.82).

While the idea behind multimethod research is relatively simple, and a logical answer to the complexities of life, its planning and execution is less straightforward. Unlike the academic researcher who selects problems that are theoretically challenging, the researcher within a management setting is asked to solve actual problems. The researcher, then, has to match the empirical problem with his or her own theoretical orientation and research style. More often than not responding with the choice of one research style is inadequate, and researchers have two options: to collaborate with researchers who employ different methods, or to combine within their own research design methods that integrate different theoretical perspectives in order to provide explanations.

The reality of health service research is that problems tend to be presented by managers and policy makers. However, the way in which these problems are formulated are not necessarily researchable, and the translation into a research problem is the researcher's first task. This also opens up opportunities to refine or re-orientate the question into one with both pragmatic and theoretical value. The latter is important if health services research is to develop, and not be confined to the problems of the day. The development of concepts that have general and longer term value stimulates management thinking, and research projects should have this dual purpose.

Managers and researchers have to reach a common understanding of the problem before strategies for data collection are agreed. Managers often are important gatekeepers to the research sites (Alaszewski and Ong, 1990), and as such need to have a grasp of the nature and objectives of the research. In multimethod research a variety of managers, grassroots staff and users of services could be involved in the data gathering process. Access to these different populations or locations has to be cleared in accordance with the specific method chosen for each site. For example, if secondary data analysis on a ward consists of examining care plans in order to assess the impact of primary nursing on patient recovery, nursing managers (operational and educational) and all nursing staff have to be aware of this objective, and collaborate through making information available.

In multimethod research data collection through different methods can have two aims: either to achieve comparability, that is, the different sets of data obtained by each method actually refer to the same problem; or to achieve contrast, whereby theoretical imagination can be triggered by contrasting data that describe a wide range of natural variation. The consequence is that the greater the variety of empirical findings to be explained, the fewer are the possible hypotheses (Brewer and Hunter, 1989).

Hakim (1987) notes that multimethod research is already common practice in policy and market research, which emphasizes the production of valid and reliable conclusions to provide a firm basis for action. In order to deliver this sort of outcome, methodological triangulation is a necessary requirement. This rather jargonized term refers to multiple measurement which tries to pinpoint the values of a phenomenon more accurately by sighting in on it from different methodological viewpoints (Brewer and Hunter, 1989, p.17). Basically the researcher infers validity from agreement between data sets which are collected through different methodologies. Theoreticians distinguish between four types of triangulation (Denzin quoted in Hakim, 1987), but the most important issue is the fact that multimethod research aims to heighten confidence in the findings of each method, because the findings converge despite the methods' differences (Brewer and Hunter, 1989, p.165). Thus, the importance of designing an appropriate research study for the problem at hand cannot be overestimated if the different methods are to effectively complement each other.

Managers make decisions about doing or commissioning research, and a cost-benefit analysis is an important element in that process. In this analysis time, financial costs and outcomes are the main factors to be considered. On the face of it multimethod research appears to be lengthy, costly and complex in its interpretation. Arguments in favour of this approach have to take account of these considerations.

Brewer and Hunter (1989) identify the costs of different methods: participant observation involves few costs to the research subjects, but requires intensive involvement of researchers; in survey and experimental research subjects have to invest time and commitment, to be matched by researchers' effort in recruiting people for the study, and in collecting data. In short, Brewer and Hunter argue that there are two types of costs: gathering data and generating data. When doing multimethod research these two types of costs will most probably be incurred, but not necessarily in a cumulative fashion. For example, in an evaluation study of a residential unit for children with severe learning difficulties, Alaszewski and Ong (1990) carried out an observation study and simultaneously used 'slack' research times (for example, when the children were at school) to examine records and other secondary data sources. Thus, the costs were not those of observation plus secondary data analysis, but of observation with reduced secondary data time.

Managers will find it important to estimate the extent to which economies can be made within multimethod research, whilst generating more in depth and complete coverage of the subject matter. This means that quality of research design and expected outcome has to be gauged against direct research costs. There is no exact measurement of this trade-off but past experience of researchers in this field can give some indication of the balance between the two variables, and the overall benefit of the multimethod approach.

CASE 1   ASSESSING THE NEEDS OF THE OVER 75-YEAR-OLD POPULATION IN
GENERAL PRACTICE

The background

The 1990 GP contract (DoH, 1989) specifies that all patients aged 75 or over have to be offered a yearly assessment of their needs. These needs are considered to fall within the social, mobility, sensory, continence, general functional and medication areas, and to take place within the person's home environment. For GPs it is therefore essential to have an accurate understanding of the number of over-75 year old people in their practice population, and then assess the various aspects of need in order to deploy the practice resources effectively and efficiently to meet those needs. A methodology capable of combining these two elements is a chief requirement for GPs and health service managers if the objectives of the 1990 contract are to be met.

The concept of need

The White Papers *Working for Patients* (DoH, 1989b) and *Caring for People* (DoH, 1989a) both assume that we can assess need as expressed in the use of health services, or through proxy measures such as indicators of deprivation. There appears to be considerable underlying confusion of what constitutes need, and the dominant political view conflates need with expressed need, that is, a felt need as expressed in a demand for an existing service. By taking expressed need as a basis for needs assessment various complications arise: is need expressed because there is a felt need or because a particular service is on offer? Do people ask for advice or treatment because they are urged to do so by professionals or social networks, for example, asking for dietary advice from the GP because of social pressure to lose weight, rather than because the individual perceives it as a need? Does demand reflect real need, or differential access to services?

There are also a number of theoretical perspectives on need. Philosophers concentrate on the role of need in bringing out what is *vital* (original emphasis) to human beings in questions of the distribution of benefits and burdens (Wiggins and Dermen, 1987). Doyal and Gough (1991) attempt to formulate a theory of human need and claim that 'since physical survival and personal autonomy are the preconditions for any individual action in any culture, they constitute the most basic human needs – those which must be satisfied to some degree before actors can effectively participate in their form of life to achieve any other valued goals' (p.54).

Sociologists rely on Bradshaw's taxonomy of need which makes the following distinctions: normative need as externally defined by 'experts'; felt need which is a perceived need or want; expressed need is a need turned into action as a demand; comparative need, which is obtained by the identification of the characteristics of the population in receipt of a service and subsequent definition of those with similar characteristics not in receipt as 'in need' (Bradshaw, 1972). Health economists focus on the idea that needs are relative and can be traded off against each other. They argue against the notion of subjectivity in needs assessment as it is open to manipulation, and propose to measure a reduction in need rather than total need. In effect, this means a measurement of changes in the benefits and costs of providing more or less of different forms of health care, i.e. marginal costs and marginal benefits of health care. They consider that with limited resources a cost-effectiveness analysis is an important management tool (Donaldson and Mooney, 1991; Sculpher and Buxton, 1991). Epidemiologists examine the measurement of health status as a determinant of need, and public health has a tradition of focusing on inequality in health which provides indication of the extent of unmet or unequally met need (RUHBC, 1989; Jacobson *et al.*, 1991).

Increasingly, health service managers have opted for a pragmatic definition of need, namely as the ability to benefit in some way from health care (Stevens and Gabbay, 1991). They argue that the ability of a population to benefit from health care depends on: firstly, the number of individuals affected, that is the incidence and prevalence of the condition under question; secondly, the effectiveness of the services available to deal with it. However, the problem is that many needs cannot be easily demarcated as health care needs, nor are people reducible to conditions, but rather to a set of conditions which determine their need for health. In managerial terms, the Stevens and Gabbay model provides conceptual handles for the contracting process, but is insufficient for understanding complex needs of populations, or specific client groups.

Given this multitude of theoretical perspectives, no one methodology can capture the complexity of need, and the multimethod approach to the measurement of need appears to be the most logical answer. Furthermore, this multimethod approach has to embrace the idea of multidisciplinary assessment, as each of the above mentioned theoretical frameworks is derived from different disciplines. The strengths and weaknesses of each approach have to be assessed in order to arrive at a research design capable of answering the question of need and the allocation of resources.

The research design

The Department of Health provided a grant for a project to be administered by Cheshire FHSA, supported by a Steering Group consisting of the Regional Advisor for General Practice, the Community Services Manager from the DHA and an outside resource person from the London School of Hygiene and Tropical Medicine. The objective of the project was to produce a documented model for use in the assessment of needs and the allocation of resources for the health care of the over-75-year-old population of three general practices in the Crewe Health District. The research was put out for tender, and a multidisciplinary team was awarded the contract (Paton *et al.*, in progress).

The research falls into two parts and the project is designed accordingly with first, the assessment of the needs of the over-75 population in the three practices and second, the analysis of the management of resources.

Part 1 Needs assessment

The assessment of need aims to assess the incidence and prevalence of specific problems related to old age. Incidence refers to the number of new cases of disease in a defined population over a particular time, and is often expressed as an annual rate. Prevalence is the number of persons with a disease in a given population at a specified point, and is usually expressed as a rate, called the point prevalence rate (Buchan *et al.*, 1990).

At present people over 75 years of age consume more health and social services than those aged between 65 and 74 (Thane, 1989). However, this pattern is not static, and when examining trends over time, one can detect improvements in health of the population as a whole, including older people. This means that in the future the over-75 population will not necessarily place a heavy burden on health and social services (compare this to the situation of a hundred years ago when people were considered old in their fifties). It has, furthermore, been argued that biological ageing does not automatically lead to ill health and dependency, because this is largely determined by cultural factors such as the values and expectations of society.

Finch (1986) puts forward a more general argument about age groupings: 'first, age groups, however constituted, should not be treated as if they have some autonomous and lasting significance outside the particular social and economic contexts which give them meaning. Second, researchers should always make explicit their own assumptions about the age categories whether they are intended simply as numerical categories, or whether they are meant to reflect meaningful age groupings in the social world. Third, where age groupings are intended to be socially meaningful, their meaning should be demonstrated rather than assumed, and related to the specific social, economic and political contexts from which that meaning derives' (p.19).

This argument is important in the present study, where the banding of the over-75 group is based on epidemiological evidence of increasing numbers in this age group with an increase in the burden of ill health. Furthermore, this banding is directly related to the consumption of health and social services resources; for example, about 50% of all hospital beds are occupied by this age group (Thane, 1989). Because the research project was managerially driven the parameters for the age grouping were set by this way of thinking. Of course, this is not unrelated to dominant cultural values which a priori consider people over 75 years of age as infirm.

In the light of the social and biological determination of old age measuring the incidence and prevalence of disease becomes important, as it attempts to provide a more objective view of the state of ill health of a defined group of people. At the same time, many measures rely on people's self-assessment of ill health, and these are equally bounded by cultural frames of reference. Furthermore, self-reporting tends to underestimate disease which is clinically defined (Blaxter, 1990). Despite these caveats, studies based on self-report form an important source of information.

Secondary analysis

The study uses two major data sets. The first one is the Health and Lifestyle Survey (Cox, *et al.*, 1987), which provides evidence that, as in many other health studies, it is the relative prevalence of disease and disability which most characterizes ageing (Blaxter, 1990, p.52). At all ages women were more likely than men to report illness, with the period between 45 and 59 being the one of poorest health. This survey produced important health status data which could be re-analysed for the over-75 population in order to provide indications for the levels of prevalence to be expected in the Crewe study.

The main measures were:

- disease and impairment or their absence, based on reported medically defined conditions and the degrees of disability which accompany them;
- experienced illness or freedom from illness, based on reports of symptoms suffered;
- psycho-social malaise or well-being, based on reports of psycho-social symptoms (Blaxter, 1990, p.42).

The second data set came from the OPCS study on the prevalence of disability among adults (Martin *et al.*, 1988). Tapes with the original data were purchased through the ESRC data archive. The tapes, written in SPSS export format, were re-analysed on a mainframe computer using SPSSX.

The significance of this study lies in the fact that many disabilities are caused by impairments that arise as a consequence of the ageing process. The survey found that the overall rate of disability rises with age, and particularly steeply after the age of 70. Almost half of the disabled adults were aged 70 years or over. Furthermore, the very elderly (80 and over) predominate among the most severely disabled adults, i.e. 41% in the two highest severity categories (Martin *et al.*, 1988, p. xii). Considering these findings it seemed appropriate to re-analyse the data for the Crewe study population in order to estimate patterns of disability, and draw comparisons with the national sample. An important limitation of the OPCS survey is that reliable results can be obtained at regional level, but below that considerable caution has to be applied in interpretation.

The secondary analysis of the above two surveys has as its main advantage that they are based on samples which cannot easily be surpassed in scope, size and quality (Dale *et al.*, 1988). The survey material from the two studies can provide an indication of the extent and distribution of disease and disability in the over-75 population, and serve as a comparative background to the Crewe study.

The next area for secondary analysis is the examination of service uptake data. This will provide indications of the extent to which expressed needs are met, and by which service provider. As Stevens and Gabbay (1991) note, this can indicate either that need, demand and supply overlap in a perfect fit, or that demand and supply coincide, where a need is not necessarily present. In order to separate out these two situations, a self-assessment and professional assessment of need has to be made, which can demonstrate the existence of discrepancies between need, demand and supply. This issue will be addressed at a later stage.

The main databases to be interrogated are the GP based computerized age–sex register, and over-75 screenings; community based Comway 2000 system which can give information on client assessments, interventions and treatments (by professional group, most notably district nurses, chiropodists, occupational therapists, CPNs); hospital referral data from those hospitals which are contracted to provide services; Social Services data available through the CRISS system (most importantly, occupational therapy and team for the elderly) and any data held by voluntary organizations.

Survey and sampling frame

The three participating practices together have approximately 3000 people over the age of 75 on their list. A survey has been carried out assessing people's overall health status, their functional ability, social networks and use of services. This provided a picture of health and health care needs, which will feed into the second step of the research project.

Instead of dividing the total population into subgroups. for example, people with physical disabilities, people with no apparent health problems, people with early Alzheimer's disease, etc., the sample has been drawn from the total practice list of over-75-year-old persons. The aim of the project is to provide the practices with a model which can assist them with the identification of the 'at risk' person, rather than to examine in depth a specific type of client. Thus, a 10% random sample, i.e. 300 people (100 from each practice), was drawn and stratified according to age (75–85 band, 85+) and sex (in order to reflect the preponderance of females).

The sample was scrutinized by a health professional so that individuals were identified who could experience difficulty in filling in a self-administered questionnaire. They were offered assistance. The other respondents received a set of questionnaires, accompanied by a letter from the practice requesting their co-operation, and a stamped addressed envelope for return to the research team.

The tools that have been selected for the study are first, the Nottingham Health Profile (Hunt *et al.*, 1986). The NHP is designed to measure perceived health problems and the extent to which such problems affect daily activities, but it is best regarded as a measure of distress in the physical, emotional and social domains. It is appropriate in many different settings, for example, to measure improvements in patients undergoing treatment for kidney stones (Mays *et al.*, 1990), as a survey tool on general populations where it can demonstrate that good health does not necessarily imply an absence of problems (Wilkin *et al.*, 1987) or as a need indicator for health planning (Bucquet and Curtis, 1986). The NHP has particular strengths as a survey tool for selected populations where there are likely to be a high proportion of scorers. As such it is highly appropriate for the over-75 client group.

The NHP is a two-part self-administered questionnaire of which Part II is optional. It is a copyrighted instrument and the schedules have to be obtained from the original designers. The areas covered by the NHP are: sleep, energy, emotional reactions, social isolation, physical mobility and pain. Bowling (1991) argues that the NHP does not focus on health, but rather on ill health – in common with many other similar instruments. The respondent is simply required to answer 'yes' or 'no' to a set of statements, according to whether it is applicable to her or his general state at the time of completing the questionnaire. It is important that the questionnaire is administered in the same manner to all respondents.

An important advantage of the NHP is that it is well accepted, and it is fully tested for validity and reliability. Numerous studies have been carried out employing this tool, and a detailed manual on its use is available.

The second instrument is the adapted Townsend Disability Scale, a concise index comprising a list of activities of daily living. Difficulties with each activity are equally scored and an aggregate (unweighted) score is calculated. The scale has proven to be acceptable to older people (Bowling, 1991) and it is its brevity which makes it easy to administer. Validity and reliability are, however, not fully tested.

Recent research (Farquhar *et al.*, 1992) has demonstrated the central importance of social networks in maintaining health in older people. Various methods exist for assessing the existence and strengths of social networks (see Wilkin *et al.*, 1992), but many involve time-consuming qualitative network analysis, using a sociometric methodology (Lundberg *et al.*, 1958) or multidimensional, complex methodologies (Wenger, 1989). Instead, the project applies a method whereby the older person him/ herself assesses the nature and importance of their social network.

The Social Support Behavioural Scale (SS-B) developed by Vaux *et al.* (1987) seeks to understand different modes of supportive behaviour given to respondents by family and friends. It has been administered to groups of students, and therefore requires some adaptation to older people. Furthermore, the length of the scale (45 items) could be reduced without losing validity as long as the balance between the different dimensions is maintained.

The SS-B contains five key dimensions of supportive behaviours including emotional, practical, financial, social and advisory support. It has demonstrated predictive value, especially in relation to psychological distress. It is, as yet, not fully tested for validity and reliability.

The above three instruments were administered to the 300 selected respondents, with an overall response rate of 77.8%. A preliminary analysis of the results has been carried out (Shiels, 1992b), but the final report will be available at the end of the project.

In addition to the needs assessment, a short index of actual service usage across health, social services and voluntary organizations was distributed. This aimed to accumulate evidence on needs which are locally met, and complemented the information gained from the social network analysis. The results form the first step in assessing the scope and performance of service provision on which the second part of the study is to elaborate.

Professional assessment

The majority of decisions about the allocation of resources are based upon the assessment of normative need, or professionally based judgements. Two methods are employed for examination of professional assessments: first, all GP screening summaries of the sample population are to be analysed, and prevalence of specific diseases and disabilities extracted. Where possible, the natural history of the disease and severity will be established. This information will be correlated with the results of the self-assessments.

Twenty five per cent of the 300 person sample, i.e. 75 individuals, will be assessed in more detail by the GP using the same indicators as the three self-assessment tools. Thus, an aggregate list will be compiled representing the dimensions of the NHP, Townsend scale and SS-B, in order to produce equivalent comparisons between normative and felt needs. Discrepancies between the two sets of assessments are important indicators for unmet need.

Part 2 Resource management

When the NHS Management Board decided to instigate the so-called resource management initiative in 1986 the stated aims were to build on the involvement of doctors and nurses in management; to bring together clinical and financial information about treatment activity; and to put clinicians and managers in a position to monitor outcomes of health care (Black, 1988). Since then, the introduction of Clinical Directorates, the purchaser–provider split and medical audit have overtaken much of what resource management tried to achieve. Yet, the underlying principles could still be applied. This is particularly true for community based health care for elderly people. Farrington (1987) argued that not only do they consume a large proportion of community services, but that the distribution of the elderly is a critical component for management of resources.

Thus, a research design has to comprise the following components:

- The formulation of a series of 'protocols' – carried out by professionals and research team using a modified Delphi technique format (Levine, 1984) – representing the agreed best response to the needs identified. This approach takes into account the purchasing framework, contrasting needs and finite human and financial resources.
- Workload analysis, providing information on all patient and non-patient related activity occurring in the Primary Health Care Team. A systematic comparison with the findings of the first part of the project will provide indicators for priority setting and 'at risk' identification, so that resources, needs and programmes of care can be optimally matched. This will also involve connecting activity information to spending and budgetary patterns.
- Development of a framework for future outcome assessment and 'optimal' use of resources, which evaluates actions against the fulfilment of identified needs. This conceptual work can form the basis for cost-effectiveness analysis.

As an example of multimethod research this project demonstrates that the weakness of secondary data analysis in not offering locally sensitive data is offset by the strengths of the battery of survey tools which incorporate subjectivity and self-assessment, but at the same time are capable of revealing local and more general patterns of health needs. The different tools selected are each focusing on different dimensions of need, and as such are capable of testing convergence.

The resource management part combines more qualitative methods such as the modified Delphi technique with pure quantitative activity analysis which, again, can be tested for convergence. As a totality, the project intends to produce a model which provides a coherent overview of the current health status of the over-75 population, and the appropriateness of the service response.

CASE 2   A MODEL OF JOINT NEEDS ASSESSMENT FOR PEOPLE WITH PHYSICAL
DISABILITIES

The background

Central to the 1989 NHS reforms are the changing roles of the DHAs and
Local Authorities, including the Social Services Departments, into
becoming 'enabling authorities'. The key feature of this role is 'to
identify needs for care among the population it serves, plan how best to
meet those needs, set overall strategies, priorities and targets, commission and purchase as well as provide necessary services and ensure their
quality and value' (DoH, 1990). In practice, the DHAs, SSDs and FHSAs
will assess the needs of populations, whilst GPs (and GP fundholders)
and Care Managers assess the needs of individuals. The emphasis of
government guidance tends to lie on the supply side as SSDs are asked to
identify 'how the care needs of individuals approaching them for
assistance will be assessed; how service needs identified following the
introduction of systematic assessment will be incorporated into the
planning process' (DoH, 1990).

In contrast, the view from the World Health Organization is that the
needs of people with disabilities are not confined to their expressed need
(or the requests for assistance). They developed a conceptual framework
which distinguishes the three elements of disablement (WHO, 1980):
impairment which is 'any loss or abnormality of psychological, physiological or anatomical structure or function'; disability as 'any restriction
or lack (resulting from an impairment) of ability to perform an activity in
the manner or within the range considered normal for a human being';
handicap is defined as 'a disadvantage for a given individual, resulting
from an impairment or disability, that limits or prevents the fulfilment of
a role (depending on age, sex and social and cultural factors) for that
individual'.

In relation to the assessment of need disability is the main concept as it
emphasizes the experience of daily life in both a functional and
psychological sense, whilst straddling health and social dimensions. It
focuses on how the individual defines her or his own disabilities and
their impact. Any model of needs assessment has to understand both the
prevalence of symptoms of disease and its disabling consequences. It
follows that this assessment is broader than analysing 'requests for
assistance' and, of necessity has to be multidisciplinary and multi-
agency. The care management approach, to some extent, accepts this
viewpoint, but the needs assessments of populations continue to be
largely unidimensional, either health or social services oriented.

Against this background Mersey Regional Health Authority's Priority
Services Department commissioned a research project which was aimed

at the production of a model for joint needs assessment across DHAs, FHSAs and SSDs, using the client group of people with physical disabilities as a case example.

The research design

The first stage of the project was to make an inventory of needs assessment approaches in the region, and compare their methodologies with national demonstration projects. Any models of good practice that were identified could be highlighted and disseminated across the region. Thus, the objective for this part of the project was to describe:

- projects aimed at assessing the needs of specific client groups or populations;
- projects which integrated work across different organizations;
- models for joint needs assessment.

Following from this exercise, one site would be selected for developmental work to develop the model for joint needs assessment.

The methodology employed for this inventory was very straightforward: interviewing key personnel from the three organizations in all the districts within the region, and a small selection of voluntary organizations active in policy formulation and service planning. Interviews were unstructured, that is, they followed a thematic format but allowed for detailed answers by the respondents. Notes were made during the interviews, and later analysed according to the main themes of the definition of need and needs assessment models, information systems, collaboration, user involvement and work on specific client groups.

SSDs tended to focus on model building for care management and individual needs assessment. Collaboration with DHAs and FHSAs was often good at locality/neighbourhood levels, but less explicit at senior management level. Furthermore, the responsibility for the implementation of the *Caring for People* targets was seen to lie firmly with SSDs. FHSAs involvement in needs assessment was uneven, with some moving towards a shared database with SSDs and DHAs, while others carried out small ad hoc projects. In DHAs the pressures for assessing demand and supply outweighed the concern with overall needs assessment. Most approaches were directly tied to the contracting process, and emphasis was placed on collecting disease-specific information. Some voluntary organizations used the OPCS disability survey data to estimate levels of need in their area. However, they were mainly concerned with safeguarding existing resources (as they largely depend on grants) and building on those to meet increasing demand.

There is a dearth of national projects concerned with joint needs assessment. Barking and Havering DHA and FHSA have set up a unified purchasing project with the aim of rapidly improving primary and community services, progressing unification of commissioning and giving an innovative lead on integrated purchasing. One of the key activities of the project is needs assessment, focusing on localities and building a model capable of priority setting. A similar project has been described for Bromley (Dean *et al.*, 1992).

The second project is based at the Public Health Research and Resource Centre in Salford, aimed at applying a public health approach to needs assessment and contracting. A case study on visual impairment amongst older people will focus on the identification of both medically defined and subjectively perceived needs. The approach involves an examination of quality, outcome and identification of service options through intersectoral collaboration. Secondary data analysis, a local survey on self-perceived needs, and vision tests form the research design. The project hopes to formulate a model which can relate information needs on consumer views to the development of contracts.

The pilot project

On the basis of the two examples and the inventory of the region a pilot project was formulated in September 1991, which was to take place in Northwich, Cheshire. The preconditions in this site were favourable: there were established and good working relationships between the three statutory agencies, and some contacts with voluntary bodies and self-help groups. A steering group with managers from all three organizations was set up to define the project with the researchers, and to ensure that it continued to be of relevance to policy and service planning. It was agreed that the choice of people with physical disabilities was appropriate for the project as it intended to develop a methodology to jointly assess needs of a particular client group, with the capability of being applied to other client groups.

The subsidiary objectives were defined as follows:

- to provide an estimate of the prevalence of physical disability in the Northwich population;
- to provide an overview of the different needs of the people identified as having physical disabilities;
- to evaluate the pattern of service delivery and make recommendations for improving service provision.

A number of users were involved in the first phase of the project. They helped formulate key issues for consideration, gave an overview of important self-help initiatives (for example, the Access group had targeted a number of public premises to be improved) and gave feedback on project activities. Yet, the project was predominantly organization-led, because the main aim was to stimulate joint needs assessment between statutory organizations and to develop a model to facilitate managerial decision-making.

Step 1 The target group

The steering group defined the target group in accordance with the OPCS disability study (Martin *et al.*, 1988), namely adults between 16 and 60 years of age. The same categories covering physical disability were used (and which are included in the ICIDH): problems with locomotion, stretching and reaching, dexterity, seeing, hearing, personal care, continence, communication (speech problems). Furthermore, the same accommodation categories were included, namely people living in private housing and those in residential accommodation. In consultation with professionals working in the Northwich area exact geographical boundaries were determined.

Step 2 The definition of need

The earlier discussion of case 1 has already outlined the philosophical underpinning of the concept of need. It suffices to state that a two-fold definition of need is used in this study: first, felt need which is considered to mean 'wants', covering the health and social arenas. Thus, it measures the experience of disability, both of individuals and groups, and the ways in which they want this to be alleviated. Second, care need, whereby need is defined as what people can benefit from. This generally includes service responses which are varied, and subject to negotiation.

Both types of need encompass met and unmet need, requiring a multimethod approach. As in the study described in case 1 the OPCS disability survey data can be re-analysed to provide a comparative background, and indicators for expected levels of prevalence.

Step 3 Developing concepts

The OPCS disability study served as a guide for assessing the impact of disability on people and the concepts employed in this study are described in detail in the report. The developmental work for the questionnaires was based on the Lambeth survey of disability (Patrick and Peach, 1989) and augmented with adaptations and innovations. The production of the measures of severity of disability passed through five stages, involving professionals, people with disabilities and carers, and voluntary organizations. Without going into the technical details of using judges to arrive at severity weightings, the important point to make is that the OPCS disability survey is grounded in the experience of disability, and as such takes into account qualitative aspects.

Understanding the experience of services is an equally important issue, because it can provide a link between subjective health status and subjective demand for services. Locally initiated work existed from which to derive relevant concepts. In 1989/90 Cheshire SSD inspection team had designed a study aimed at eliciting information from people with physical disabilities about their experiences of local services, and their views about their unmet needs. The questionnaire used was largely open-ended as emphasis was placed upon understanding people's experiences as expressed in their own words.

The sample was drawn from the Cheshire area, but did not delineate the sampling frame in any other way. Respondents were recruited through the local media, through service channels, for example day centres and libraries, and through word-of-mouth. As such, the sample was uncontrolled and purely opportunistic. In total 585 questionnaires were filled in, many with personal letters attached. The problem of analysing this number of open-ended questionnaires was not resolved, and only 10% (randomly selected from the 585, instead of a sample stratified for age, sex and geographical location) were analysed for the inspection report (Dickenson, 1990).

For the present study all completed questionnaires from the Northwich area ($n=41$) were analysed, utilizing the method of multidimensional representation of disablement developed by Hirst (1990). This model provides a structural representation of people with the same disabilities who are then grouped together. The components are linked to form a lattice which displays an overview of the different levels of disability. In this way the lattice provides a complete classification of mutually shared disabilities by revealing all the interrelationships between individuals and their disablement experience.

In the Northwich sample only two levels emerged (in contrast to Hirst who arrived at four levels). This does not imply that the disablement experience in Northwich is of a less complex character, but rather that the data collected was not primarily intended to examine the different layers of experience. Thus, the Northwich data only allowed for a limited analysis.

An important caveat is that the Northwich sample is predominantly drawn from people who attend the local day centre. It is not known why the survey has not been able to attract other people from the area to respond to the questionnaire (this is in sharp contrast with, for example, Chester). As a result, the sample is skewed to a particular type of service user, which could explain the relative 'flatness' of the lattice (Figure 7.1).

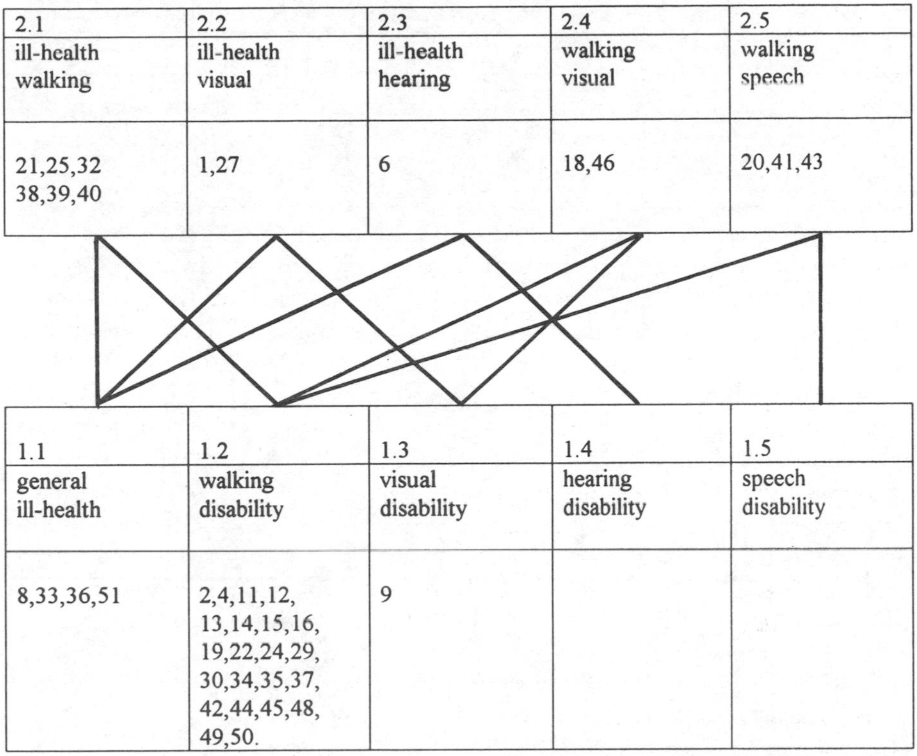

2.1	2.2	2.3	2.4	2.5
ill-health walking	ill-health visual	ill-health hearing	walking visual	walking speech
21,25,32 38,39,40	1,27	6	18,46	20,41,43

1.1	1.2	1.3	1.4	1.5
general ill-health	walking disability	visual disability	hearing disability	speech disability
8,33,36,51	2,4,11,12, 13,14,15,16, 19,22,24,29, 30,34,35,37, 42,44,45,48, 49,50.	9		

Note: the numbers in the boxes denote respondent numbers

Figure 7.1 Lattice representation of experience of physical disability

As expected, the people suffering from mobility problems constitute the largest group, and the combination of general ill health with mobility problems is most common amongst the more complex client group.

When analysing service usage it is clear that, by virtue of having been assessed as suitable for day centre care, individuals are able to access a range of other services. Looking more closely at the clients with more complex needs (i.e. level 2) it becomes evident that they are in receipt of at least one other service (Table 7.1).

The main area of concern emerging from this analysis is transport, which is also highlighted in the inspection report. The analysis demonstrates that transport is not necessarily distributed according to need. Self-help groups consider this a key issue for social integration, which research has shown is an important predictor of well-being in chronic illness (Fitzpatrick *et al.*, 1991). Furthermore, access to suitable and affordable transport has been well-established as a key prerequisite to uptake of services.

Multimethod research

Table 7.1 Level of client's difficulties, by service

Level	Number	DC	SW	DN	VO	HC	TR	PH	OT	SP	RE
2.1	21	1	1	1	1						
	25		1	1	1	1	1				
	32	1	1	1				1			
	38	1	1	1			1		1		
	39		1		1						
	40	1		1				1	1		
2.2	1	1	1							1	
	27	1	1								
2.3	6	1	1				1				1
2.4	18	1							1		
	46	1	1	1			1				
2.5	20	1				1			1	1	
	41	1	1							1	
	43		1								

Key:
DC day centre
SW social worker
DN District Nurse
VO voluntary organization
HC home care

TR transport
PH physiotherapy
OT occupational therapy
SP speech therapy
RE respite care

This particular subsample reports very little in the way of unmet need, which is logical considering the high level of service input. It therefore provides evidence that one key service opens the door for accessing other provisions. In terms of the experience of disability it illustrates a structured pattern, if less complex than that of the Hirst study.

The SSD study helped to define what (potential) users perceived as key service issues. The classification of the open-ended questions facilitated the formulation of a list of services within the area that were either provided or would be desirable. In this way, indirect user involvement assisted with the development of a service profile for testing in a wider survey.

Survey and sampling frame

The concepts derived from the OPCS disability survey and the SSD survey formed the backbone for the development of a structured questionnaire to be administered through a survey. If an overview of needs and an evaluation of service provisions was to be achieved, a survey demonstrating prevalence and describing the experience of disablement in Northwich was required. The target group for a survey contained two types of possible respondents:

1. people known to the statutory agencies;
2. people not known to the statutory agencies.

Different strategies for reaching each of these groups had to be employed.

Group 1

The Access group advised on methods to find people who are not in contact with statutory services. Four possible avenues were indicated:

1. accessing people through the registers kept by various self-help groups. This could give access to people using and not using statutory services;
2. contacting people through the voluntary organizations network;
3. inviting people to participate in the study, that is, through a process of self-selection. First, a similar strategy to the SSD survey was used, asking people to react to articles in the local media. With the backing of a county councillor two Northwich based papers ran features explaining the project, and invited people who considered themselves as physically disabled to come forward to answer the questionnaire. Second, posters were displayed in Local Authority and health service buildings, asking the same question as the newspaper articles. The response to these two strategies has been extremely limited, with the main problem being the inability to estimate the potential response;
4. drawing a sample from registers such as the Orange Badge scheme. The main problem, however, is that these registers are broad, including a wide diversity of people, which makes it difficult to focus on those who fit the criteria of the study.

Group 2

Drawing a sample from people known to the service has been done through each of the three statutory agencies. Three subsamples were compiled:

1. Through the SSD computerized register of occupational therapy, 260 cases (1990–1991), of which 36 were open cases, were identified. Two hundred and fourteen of these were classed as chronically sick and disabled, with small numbers in the categories of deaf, deaf without speech, hard of hearing, blind, partially sighted people. A further six people had more than one registered disability.

A 20% sample was drawn from the group of chronically sick and disabled people, while the remaining categories were included in total. Thus, the overall SSD sample was 88 respondents.

The SSD wrote letters to all 88 people, explaining the study and asking for people's collaboration. The questionnaires were then sent out by the research team, with a covering letter and stamped addressed reply envelope.

2. The second subsample was based on the District Nurses' caseload, whereby the District Nurses selected names from their handheld records, following the same criteria as the SSD sampling. After cross-checking with the SSD sample, two people were deleted from this subsample. A total of 25 names was generated, and the nurses distributed the questionnaires themselves, with the covering letter from the research team and stamped addressed envelope.

3. The FHSA has no centrally based system for drawing client population samples. GP age–sex registers are not suitable unless individual GPs have inserted special codes for people with physical disabilities. One GP offered to collaborate on a pilot basis, and selected nine people from his own list who had physical disabilities but were not in receipt of services from SSD or DHA. It is interesting to speculate upon the possibilities this avenue opens up in assessing unmet need, because if Peach and Patrick (1989) are right GPs are the formal service most frequently used by people with disabilities.

There are examples of detailed scientific policy oriented research such as the Lambeth study (Patrick and Peach, 1989), but this type of costly enterprise cannot be replicated by health services managers who have to assess needs on a yearly basis. It is, therefore, important to use the in-depth studies as guiding and background material, but design studies which are local, flexible and topical.

The multimethod approach chosen here exploits the analysis of secondary data to the full, and uses qualitative work to formulate concepts. The survey is then capable of testing these concepts on a wider range of people, and providing a disability profile based on users of different services. The more experimental and less controlled methods of recruiting respondents through the media warrant further exploration, but should be developed for client groups with fluid boundaries. They are premised upon people's own perception of their identity as someone with or without disabilities, which crucially determines their demand for services.

The study design is schematically represented in Figure 7.2.

Selected survey results

The self-administered postal questionnaire contained questions about problems with mobility, seeing, hearing, personal care, continence, pain,

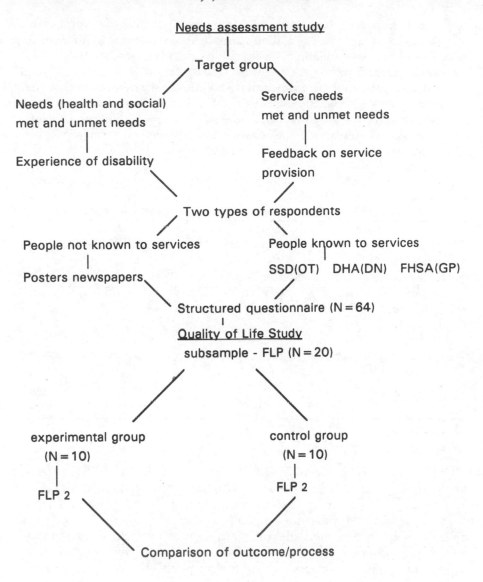

Figure 7.2 Study design

availability and use of services. The Social Services sample (88) and the GP sample (9) together yielded a 66% response rate (64), while the organization of the Community Nursing sample failed. The analysis of the results is, therefore, based solely on the returns of the SSD and GP sample.

Because the number of people responding is relatively small, a breakdown into each individual item is of limited use. Therefore, a cumulative approach has been adopted which counts the number of disabilities people have, and then provides comparisons with service usage. This cross-tabulation appears to deliver more managerially relevant information.

The maximum number of physical disabilities that are measured in the questionnaire is six (3a, 3b, 3c, 3d, 3e, 3f). These dimensions were set against the following services: physiotherapy, occupational therapy, aids and adaptations, transport, social work and district nursing (see Table 7.2).

Table 7.2 Physical disability and receipt of physiotherapy services

Number of disabilities	Physiotherapy service		
	No	Yes	Total
2	1	3	4
3	5	1	6
4	2	8	10
5	3	5	8
6	9	5	14
	20	22	42
	47.6%	52.4%	100%

Of the people with disabilities (there was no score of 1), 52.4% receive physiotherapy services, while 47.6% do not. Whilst there is no clear pattern in the relationship between number of disabilities and service delivery, it is striking that nine people who report to have six physical disabilities do not receive any physiotherapy. The lack of community based physiotherapy has been long recognized, but very few districts have built up strong services outside the hospitals. The comparison with occupational therapy is shown in Table 7.3.

The shortage of occupational therapy services is even more marked, with only 23.8% people receiving this service. Again, when looking at people who report a high level of physical disability, the lack of provision is inescapable. It can be noted, for example, that none of the ten people with four disabilities receive support, either from Social Services or Health Unit based OTs. The dearth of provisions for aids and adaptations is illustrated in Table 7.4. Thus, only 21.4% of the people who report to suffer with physical disability have aids and adaptations in the

Table 7.3 Physical disability and the receipt of occupational therapy

	Occupational therapy		
Number of disabilities	No	Yes	Total
2	3	1	4
3	5	1	6
4	10	0	10
5	2	6	8
6	12	2	14
	32	10	42
	76.2%	23.8%	100%

Table 7.4 Physical disability and delivery of aids and adaptations

	Aids and adaptations		
Number of disabilities	No	Yes	Total
2	4	0	4
3	6	0	6
4	9	1	10
5	5	3	8
6	9	5	14
	33	9	42
	78.6%	21.4%	100%

home. Service providers themselves have repeatedly drawn attention to the importance of this service, but have generally been unable to achieve higher levels of input. This is borne out by the above findings, where, for example, the nine people with six disabilities have no aids or adaptations.

The first survey carried out by the Social Services Department flagged the importance of transport. This was reinforced by the Access group, who argued that in order to stimulate social integration people with disabilities should be able to get about. The results on the utilization of transport such as Dial-a-ride are not very encouraging when considering the pivotal role of transport for improving people's quality of life (Table 7.5). The implications for people who have multiple physical disabilities but who do not have access to transport are enormous, and their social

Table 7.5 Physical disability and access to transport

| Number of disabilities | Transport | | |
	No	Yes	Total
2	4	0	4
3	3	3	6
4	10	0	10
5	6	2	8
6	10	4	14
	33	9	42
	78.6%	23.4%	100%

isolation is immeasurable. In some areas voluntary organizations have developed transport schemes, but the findings from this study demonstrate that the issue requires concerted action across a variety of agencies.

Social work and district nursing input was measured, and is summarized in Tables 7.6 and 7.7.

The need for social work support and district nursing is very variable among people with physical disabilities, and the results require a supplementary assessment of the nature of their needs. For example, the results appear to illustrate the small number of people receiving district nursing care; however, many people with physical disabilities are not ill and do not need this service.

The number of vision problems recorded were at most two (3g and 3h). People with vision problems mainly used social work services, rather than any other services. The following table demonstrates that well over half of the people with vision problems have used social work support (Table 7.8).Three out of 22 people with vision problems had home care support, one person received district nursing and one had night nursing care.

Hearing problems were measured through items 3i, 3j and 3l. As with the above mentioned client group the service most frequently called upon was social work, whilst only three of the 34 people reporting hearing difficulties used district nursing services, and four had some form of home care support. (Table 7.9).

General illness was measured through five items (4a, 4b, 4c, 4d, 5b). Night nursing was used by only one person out of 42, and home care by three people. It was expected that with the general illness index the number of people receiving district nursing care would be higher than just under 20%, and it is necessary to examine the combination of problems in order to gauge why more nursing involvement has not been achieved. The social work input was slightly higher at 26%.

Table 7.6 Physical disability and social work services

| Number of disabilities | Social work | | |
	No	Yes	Total
2	4	0	4
3	5	1	6
4	9	1	10
5	4	4	8
6	9	5	14
	31	11	42
	73.8%	26.2%	100%

Table 7.7 Physical disability and district nursing

| Number of disabilities | District nursing | | |
	No	Yes	Total
2	3	1	4
3	4	2	6
4	9	1	10
5	5	3	8
6	13	1	14
	34	8	42
	80.9%	19.1%	100%

The issue of transport has already been highlighted, and is reinforced by the findings concerning the people who report difficulty in going outside (caused by a range of problems) and who have access to transport. Seventeen out of 23 people (73.9%) do not have the use of transport. At the same time 20 out of 23 (86.9%) state that they receive mobility allowance, which presumably pays for private transport. Yet, taken together there appears to be evidence that unmet needs in transport are significant.

Concerning incontinence, service uptake was very limited, with none out of 18 people who lacked bladder control using linen services, and three (16.6%) using personal hygiene services. The figures for the 13

Table 7.8 Vision problems and social work

| Number of difficulties | Social work | | |
	No	Yes	Total
1	5	4	9
2	5	8	13
	10	12	22
	45.4%	54.6%	100%

Table 7.9 Hearing difficulties and social work

| Number of difficulties | Social work | | |
	No	Yes	Total
1	7	4	11
2	11	3	14
3	5	4	9
	23	11	34
	67.6%	32.4%	100%

people who reported lack of bowel control were again 0 and 2 respectively.

On the whole, no clear pattern can be detected of when and why people utilize particular services, but overall there appear to be large areas of unmet need which require further examination and management action across different agencies.

Quality of life

As part of the current debate about the contribution of health care to human life, the notion of quality of life has gained in significance. Yet, Megone (1990) argues that the notion of quality of life has been discussed throughout the history of philosophy, and can be traced back to Aristotle. He questions the empirical and economic inspired conceptualizations on the grounds that they implicitly employ evaluative assumptions without making clear what these are. He proposes to base the quality of life debate on the Aristotelian concept which places the human capacity to reason at the centre of the quality of life. This, by extension, grounds the assessment of quality of life in fixed components determining human nature, and its evaluation base.

These ideas are very compelling, but as yet no measures have been developed on the basis of this philosophical approach. Bowling (1991) and Wilkin *et al.* (1992) review the theoretical and empirical attempts to measure quality of life and, not surprisingly, conclude that a wide diversity exists, alongside theoretical confusion and methodological inaccuracy. At the same time, continued testing of different methods remains essential in order to be able to use the concept of quality of life in health service management.

In relation to the assessment of the quality of life of people with physical disability two tools appear to promise potentially interesting results, namely the Sickness Impact Profile and the UK adaptation, the Functional Limitations Profile (Patrick and Peach, 1989). Despite their length (the FLP contains 136 items) the tools appear to be well accepted, and can be used as outcome measures for health care evaluation. They can be applied to people with chronic illness in a variety of settings, and have proven properties of reliability and validity. In this study the choice has been made to use the FLP as an outcome measure.

In the present study one key question has to be addressed, namely the underlying assumption that joint assessment and resulting joint action between DHAs, FHSAs and SSDs are more beneficial than the separate operation of the different organizations. Hudson (1990) warns that this assumption has not been proven, but that it still informs all current policy on joint working. Therefore, it is important to test whether joint approaches to care actually improve people's quality of life, and this study intends to examine this issue.

The design for the study involves the selection of an experimental and a control group from the sample surveyed in the first stage. The groups will be matched for sex, age and level of disability. All individuals in the group will receive the interviewer-administered FLP. The experimental group will receive support jointly planned by DHA, FHSA and SSD, following a care management approach, while the control group will (for six months) not receive this integrated approach to care but continue with the care pattern already provided. After six months the FLP will again be administered to all respondents in order to ascertain any change in the quality of life, and whether there is any significant difference between the two groups.

The findings are important for managers who require evidence that deploying resources in a different manner, that is, by operating a care management approach, is warranted by an improvement of the recipient's quality of life. There is, of course, a risk that the research findings do not support the change of policy, which then has to open up a discussion about the approach to care, and the roles and responsibilities of the various agencies involved. Yet, this is a risk worth taking if it results in policies which are founded on scientific evidence, rather than on belief.

CONCLUSION

It has become increasingly apparent that the complex issues facing health policy makers and health service managers cannot be addressed by relying on a single research method. Research design has to be flexible and innovative in order to examine the full scale of contemporary problems. The multimethod approach appears to be an effective response because it is capable of combining different methodologies in ways that offset strengths and weaknesses against each other, producing a multilayered analysis.

The two examples not only combine multiple methods, but are designed in different stages, where different methods are adopted in order to answer specific questions at each juncture of the research process. Thus, careful planning and intermediate analysis which assist in designing the next phase are essential steps. At the same time, a certain amount of flexibility is possible because of regular assessment and the reliance on a range of methodological tools. These characteristics make this methodological approach to design eminently suitable to the management enterprise. A continuous dialogue between researchers and managers strengthens the total process and makes the research results relevant to managerial decision-making.

Chapter Eight

Using research – the broader issues

INTRODUCTION

Underlying the discussion of the social science contribution to health service management lies the question of its use in the management enterprise. This poses two different sets of questions, namely how to define use, and to assess the generalizability of health and health care problems across varying contexts. While the emphasis in the previous chapters has been on the problems faced within developed countries, there are similarities with those encountered both in the old eastern European countries (McKee, 1991), and in the developing world (Varkevisser et al., 1990; WHO, 1988). This chapter will address some of the issues that have a more global relevance, and therefore contextualize the discussion of use, the development of strategy and the future research needs beyond the British environment.

DEFINING USE

It is not easy to recognize how and by whom social science research is used, because direct use is relatively uncommon. Very few research projects progress in a linear fashion from being commissioned through execution and completion to immediate application. Putting research results to use depends on a variety of factors, including the acceptability of the findings, whether any adaptations are needed, the policy context, available resources, etc.

Richardson et al. (1990), in their examination of research commissioned by government departments, point out that understanding the use of research is rather complex. They argue that research tends to be used in an indirect way because it serves to provide a background to decision-making rather than delivering prescriptions for change which can be immediately implemented. Thus, it is important to have a clear idea about the purpose of research, namely whether it is undertaken for its wider contribution to knowledge, or to assist with discrete and identifiable decisions – or both.

Furthermore, Richardson *et al.* demonstrate that purpose is linked to the user. The user can be a policy maker who requires research to illuminate specific issues, or a manager who wants to examine the effects of strategic or operational decisions, and so on. In order to clarify research and its application both purpose and user have to be defined at the outset for the question of use to be understood from the beginning. Richardson *et al.* also argue that resolving the question of use should precede the question of dissemination because it is essential to be clear about who might be using the research before it can be targeted appropriately.

It is interesting to note that more than a decade earlier Illsley (1980) hypothesized that the chances of implementation of research are strengthened if the research worker identifies his or her problems out of intimate knowledge of the field and its practitioners. He goes on to argue that personal contacts and ensuing discussions with practitioners and decision-makers tend to influence implementation directly.

These issues are particularly relevant when considering the contribution of social science to health services management, where the emphasis lies on the use of results. It is important to distinguish the various modes of social science research before assessing their possible 'use-value' depending on who the user is and to what purpose the research is expected to be put. The framework set out by Richardson *et al.* helps to structure the discussion on the policy relevance of social research.

DESCRIPTIVE RESEARCH

Health policy and planning require a sound understanding of the current health status of populations and their relevant social groupings. This entails an analysis of the general population and specific client or cultural groups within it, which is most commonly provided through descriptive research. In the health arena epidemiological research tends to fulfil this function, but there is considerable debate over whether this type of public health research can be value-free in its description.

Following the advent of the 'new public health' it has been argued that scientists originate from and function in society and cannot be free from ideological choices. Jacobson *et al.* state this very clearly in the introduction to their book on a strategy for health: 'We start from the position that health is important among the objectives and values of most individual human beings and that they expect their government and administrations to pursue policies that will afford them the opportunity to attain lives of optimum duration and quality' (1991, p.5). From this starting point they demonstrate that there are considerable inequalities in health between different social and cultural groupings, and that the task of policy makers is to address those inequalities. The formulation of policy should be framed by the World Health Organization's Health for All by the Year 2000 strategy, which helps to supersede the possibility that the preoccupation with competition for new resources and the use of market forces will become a substitute for policy.

As a result, this explicitly ideological stance leads to a strategy with targets aimed at influencing the determinants of disease and health which are defined numerically whenever possible. Jacobson *et al.* emphasize that most avoidable diseases have multiple causes and that each determinant of health or disease can contribute to a range of diseases. Acknowledgement of this complexity has to be reflected in a strategy by attempting to quantify only those targets for which a sufficient database exists to warrant predictions about future achievements. Other targets for action may not necessarily be quantifiable but represent areas of policy in which progress can be made.

Within this approach, descriptive epidemiological research is used to make choices in setting policy objectives and strategic targets. The underlying principle of equity has been made explicit, and as a result choices in research, at the level of both subject matter and interpretation, have been made transparent. This type of descriptive research does not consider itself as value-free, nor wishes it to be so.

The example of the Welsh health strategy demonstrates a clear link between research and policy making. In particular, the protocols for each of the ten Health Gain areas are grounded in descriptive research, while being contextualized by a strategic framework. When analysing the structure of the protocols the centrality of sound research is obvious. Each protocol starts with a detailed outline of the current position, that is, comparing the mortality and morbidity of Wales with the European region. It goes on to plot the trends, and base predictions of the future on an analysis of those trends. This leads to the identification of opportunities for health gain, and more specifically sets strategic choices for shaping the future against a resource framework, that is, assessing investment and dis-investment opportunities.

This fits into an overall approach which can be summarized as follows:

1. research on establishing the current health status of the (local) population, which results in a needs profile;
2. analysing the current and future capacity of providers in order to formulate aims and objectives for policy and strategy;
3. identifying alternative options for dealing with objectives;
4. decide on preferred options, which results in specific purchasing actions.

The above scheme illustrates the close link between research, an overarching strategy and the immediate policy environment, which operates with a split between purchasers and providers. The Welsh strategy is consistent with the HFA 2000 approach, and shows similarities with the Jacobson *et al.* model, but as it is located within the structure of the NHS, it is aligned with the dominant mode of decision-making. Therefore, the choices of research territories are determined by the strategic direction, and the descriptive analysis in the protocols is designed to enable policy formulation.

EXPLANATORY RESEARCH

The distinction between explanatory research as providing explanations for patterns of health and disease and the descriptive type as discussed above is one of gradation. In explanatory research, however, examination of the factors underlying patterning is the primary objective. The research concerned with inequalities of health (discussed in Chapter Three) focuses on explaining the reasons for inequalities, and how inequality manifests itself in health and disease.

Research influenced by anthropology attempts to illuminate the cultural factors in the epidemiology of disease. Helman (1990) argues that a range of cultural issues impinge on the perceptions of disease and illness, including family structure, gender roles, sexual behaviour, diet, housing and so on. Evidence from different societies has underlined this perspective and its significance for health planning.

For example, Nyamwaya (1987) examines the complex interrelationship between indigenous African (Pokot of Kenya) and western medicine. He demonstrates that the two paradigms can lead to complementary, competitive or supplementary explanations, which determine the use of various health services. Understanding this dynamic relationship is important for health planners in that they have to adapt their provisions so that they can respond flexibly to different needs.

The work by Herzlich (1973) has been influential within the European context. She argued that French middle-class people distinguished between illness as determined by life in an urban, advanced society, and health as determined by an individual's make-up, such as heredity, temperament, physical constitution. Such insights are important in planning services which on the one hand aim to cure disease, and on the other hand promote health. They have to be based on different logics, and take into account the wider explanations that people employ to account for their own well-being.

Similar work has been carried out within Britain, for example by Blaxter (1983), who analysed the models of disease held by poor Scottish women. Their explanations of causality were relatively complex and, while wrong in scientific detail, not necessarily unscientific. Health was defined in terms of being able to carry out their normal social roles and Blaxter demonstrated that these beliefs directly influenced health-seeking behaviour. Cornwell's research (1984) also emphasized the connection between roles and responsibilities and perceptions of being unwell. She compared male and female accounts and identified differences which related to the sexual division of labour within the household.

Both these pieces of research indicate that explanations of patterns of health and illness within and between social groups are complex, depending on an interplay of variables which are environmental, economic, social, cultural and psychological. This type of detailed research is often considered as marginal to the activity of policy-making as it has taken place within the academic context, and as such has no explicit policy objectives. Its relevance lies in posing the question whether services are responsive to the needs of populations and individuals which the research has shown to be multifaceted. Furthermore, the issue is whether services are taking into account difference and (potential) inequality in health.

STRATEGIC RESEARCH

Strategy has been variously defined as a pattern in a stream of decisions or as a pattern in a stream of actions (Mintzberg and Waters, 1990) and as a result strategic research has either concerned itself with the concept of decision and the outcomes of decision or with the links and discontinuities between decision and implementation. An example of the latter approach is the research carried out by Pettigrew *et al.* (1992) on the processes of choice and change in the NHS. They argue that frequently a gap exists between statements of intent, that is strategy, and operational implementation. In their view the decision-making process has to be considered as a continuous process in context, which means taking into account the interpretations and their variations of policy by different actors in the process.

Pettigrew *et al.* hypothesized that the rate and pace of change in the post-Griffiths NHS could be explained by a subtle interplay between the content, context and process of change. They develop a framework which distinguishes between receptive contexts for change, in which there are features of context (and management action) that seem to be favourably associated with forward movement, and non-receptive contexts which are configurations of features which may be associated with blocks to change (p.268). Based on this framework they create a multilayered analysis pinpointing key factors which can be identified and used in subsequent change processes.

The importance of this type of strategic research is that it uncovers the way an organization develops strategically by examining the various levels of decision, as well as the parts and total process. In terms of methodology such a contextual approach draws on various disciplines – and therefore various methods – in order to explain the complexity of change processes, much in the same way as research has done earlier (Hunter, as quoted in Illsley, 1980). By dissecting the connections between decision and action managers and policy makers can better understand processes of change, and forecast the implementation of strategy.

An extension of this mode is the so-called future scenarios research, which is a way of identifying key mechanisms which will affect the development of a particular field in the mid- to longer term future. The Steering Committee on Future Health Scenarios in the Netherlands has developed this type of research, and considers scenarios as an important tool for policy makers. The definition of a scenario as used within the Dutch context is: 'the description of the present state of a society, or part thereof, of possible and desirable future states, together with a series of events which could lead from the present to the future' (Van Houten quoted in Roscam Abbing, 1992).

The scenario approach explicitly links itself with policy-making because its central aim is to lay the foundation for long term policy. Within the Dutch context this type of research is carried out by specially appointed committees which formulate a scenario for the government. For example, the most recent report on public health provides an overview of the current state of the discipline within the Netherlands, followed by three scenarios which are tested on their plausibility, and are subsequently adjusted. The scenarios are then applied to two public health activities, the control of infectious diseases and public health for elderly persons. The consequences of the scenarios are worked out in terms of organizational impact, policy control, financing, information systems, expertise and effectiveness. These are then extrapolated to the full public health territory before drawing final conclusions which are to inform policy decisions.

This type of strategic research makes no apology for attempting to directly influence its use at a high level of decision-making. It is possible that because of its explicit mandate from policy makers, who define the agenda, the scenario approach meets with fewer obstacles in its implementation. Of course, it is still subject to the vagaries of the political processes surrounding policy-making, but there is a shared understanding between researchers and policy makers of the objectives and implications of the research. In that sense there is no separation between the research activity and planned service development. As such, this model is an example of what Richardson *et al.* (1990) consider to fall under the heading of direct research use.

EVALUATION RESEARCH

The methodological aspects of this type of research have already been discussed in Chapter Six, and I will therefore concentrate on the use of evaluation research. It might be expected that when evaluation is considered to be an inseparable part of service development the effect of evaluation research on policy should be a logical and direct process. In reality, this rarely happens, and Illsley (1980) has argued that there are a number of reasons for this, including ambiguity, the lack of full-scale reviews of policy, the fact that objectives vary across systems, or that changes only occur incrementally and at the margins. Most importantly, evaluation is a complex exercise, which not only includes assessing outcome and impact, but can also be concerned with understanding the nature and variability of implementation, barriers to implementation or unanticipated programme effects. Not all evaluation projects succeed in capturing this complexity, and as a result fail to make an impact on policy makers and managers.

Evaluation research has more chance to be used if it is considered as an integral part of the development process, and as such serves as a feedback loop for management. A significant departure in this field is the emergence of outcomes research. Wilkin *et al.* (1992) define outcome in the context of health and illness as the achievement of or failure to achieve desired goals. Then, outcomes can be either positive or negative, that is, ranging from complete health to death – or worse. Wilkin *et al.* focus on the primary care setting and argue that outcomes research is still relatively uncommon within that context. They feel that with the advent of medical audit a strong stimulus has emerged for the application of outcome measurement of both individual treatments in primary health care and the evaluation of patterns of service delivery (p.284). With the increasing emphasis on effectiveness and efficiency, there is strong pressure to further develop and apply outcomes research that can inform management decision-making.

Another example of a suitable arena for evaluation research is the rapidly expanding field of minimally invasive therapy. Here, health services research is concerned with evaluating effectiveness, efficiency and acceptability of innovations. Furthermore, there is increasing awareness that results have to be disseminated to managers and clinicians who are able to act on findings (Mays, in press; Advisory Group on Health Technology Assessment, 1992).

Evaluating innovations is a complex tasks which requires the input from various disciplines, as it combines the evaluation of the clinical, technical, economic, social and ethical components. Mays (in press) discusses various examples such as magnetic resonance imaging (MRI) systems which need constant upgrading in order to maintain their state of the art performance. The financial investments have to be evaluated against the question whether it will duplicate, complement or replace current imaging methods. In clinical terms does the new technology improve the accuracy of diagnosis and as a result influence patient management? From the perspective of the user one has to assess the eventual outcome and quality of life issues. In short, the evaluation resembles a cost-effectiveness analysis, while in the case of MRI the technique has been introduced before cost-effectiveness has been conclusively demonstrated. Mays concludes that this is generally the case when doctors are reasonably confident of the benefits of the new technique.

The current pressure in many health care systems has placed question marks besides examples such as the one quoted above. Medical opinion cannot be sufficient guarantee for using resources in ways that provide the most cost-effective improvement to people's health status. Evaluations should be able to address the wider consequences of implementation and therefore research should be firmly contextualized, that is, be aware of the resources available and the set of priorities which have to be weighed up against each other. The baseline for evaluation has to include the aspects mentioned by Mays, be they ethical or technical, as medical innovation does not take place in a vacuum but is part and parcel of the value system of a particular society.

DEVELOPMENTAL RESEARCH

Research using a developmental approach is geared towards progressing the discussion and implementation of service provision models. It focuses on assessing the application of theory to practice, and assists in remodelling particular approaches by a critical analysis of the interpretation and achievement of objectives. This type of research builds on a dialogue between researchers, policy makers and managers. By its very nature development research is used almost immediately.

A recent example is the work done by Leedham and Wistow (1992) on the care management approaches developed by Social Services departments, and definitions of the role of GPs in the assessment process. They carried out a review of the literature and models of good practice, conducted a telephone survey, collected detailed information in selected localities in order to provide an analysis of models. Their research contained specific recommendations for the further development of care management which were addressed both at the Department of Health and at local policy makers and practitioners. The ideas flowing from the research were founded on current care management principles, consistent with overall policy, but also offered new insights into the interpretation and extension of the basic model.

Precisely because of the above characteristics the use value of the research is great. It serves to advance the discussions between the different parties involved in the implementation of the care in the community policies. On the one hand it pushes back the boundaries of knowledge; on the other hand it remains in close contact with current practice, which means that the research can form the bridge between present and future.

METHODOLOGICAL RESEARCH

The complexity of health services management, coupled with the wide range of problems faced in health and disease, often leads to the realization that current research methodologies are inadequate in solving contemporary issues. Methodological research attempts to fill this void by testing out new methods. Its distinction from fundamental scientific research is that the need to search for new methodologies is prompted by the policy or management agenda, and close collaboration between decision makers and researchers is crucial if this type of methodological work is to be used.

A key area, which has been repeatedly referred to in this book, is needs assessment. No established methodologies exist, not least because need has been variously defined. Whether need is broadly seen as physical health and autonomy (Doyal and Gough, 1991) or as the ability to benefit from health care (Stevens and Gabbay, 1991), the science of measuring need is underdeveloped. Thus, there is a search for methodologies which are scientifically grounded and provide results which can be translated into policy and strategic management.

Depending on the theoretical underpinnings of the concept of need, methods have ranged from relying on a formal, standardized and objective measurement of need using tools that are validated and tested, to more contextual and subjective descriptions by those 'in need'. The pattern that seems to be emerging is one that combines the formal and informal assessment of need, and there is an (implicit) acknowledgement that there is no methodological consensus.

It is important for policy makers and managers to realize that the understanding of need is incomplete, largely as a result of the various theoretical perspectives on the concept of need itself, and the methodologies arising from this theoretical pluralism. At the same time, they are confronted with the reality of resource constraints, and the need to set priorities. If priorities are to be based on informed choice, needs assessment research has to be advanced. Therefore, decision makers would be well advised to work closely with researchers to progress methodological developments. The use-value of this type of research does not lie in methodological purity, but in its provision of a scientific underpinning to important choices in health care.

USING RESEARCH IN THE DEVELOPING WORLD

The six types of research discussed above are what Richardson *et al.* (1990) call policy relevant research. I have elaborated on their approach by citing examples which demonstrate how they can be used in the health policy and management context. All the examples are drawn from the developed world, but many of the issues can be extended to the developing world.

A current research priority in many developing countries is the strengthening of district health management. Most of this sort of research is instigated by development agencies who are switching from capital and revenue investment to 'capacity building' in the countries receiving assistance. The objectives of this type of research are most commonly defined in the following terms:

- to pilot approaches to improve efficiency in the utilization, allocation and delivery of resources in the health sector at district level;
- to develop replicable models which focus on increasing the efficiency of use of existing resources;
- to develop management systems and adequate training;
- to provide accessible health services to the poorest sections of the population.

In order to address this research agenda multidisciplinary teams consisting of medical doctors, economists, human resource specialists, social scientists and hospital managers adopt a multimethod research approach. This entails the collection and analysis of secondary data (e.g. utilization data, notes of meetings, planning documents), observation, interviewing and action research. A key consideration in the research is the ownership of the findings by district managers. Thus, the research strategy is built on collaboration between researchers and managers, and regular intermediate feedback.

Similarities with health management in developed countries lie in resource constraints and the pressure to demonstrate cost-effectiveness. Furthermore, there is an increasing reliance on the non-governmental sector. The main problems in many developing countries are the inadequacy of the information available, and the inappropriate use of skills at all levels. Coupled with the centralized decision-making structures this results in the lack of any effective district management.

Research into the operation of district health management and the underlying causes of its ineffectiveness has a direct impact on the allocation of resources from development agencies. It also influences strategy at district level, because many of the research findings do not necessarily require outside funding, but a re-organization of national or district management systems. For example, if the Ministry of Health genuinely devolves decision-making to district level, that is devolving budgets, district management can become a reality.

Many research findings, however, need funding. For example, the information systems are woefully inadequate. The main cause is not the lack of equipment such as computers, but the low level of understanding among the people collecting and analysing data. There is little comprehension of what data can be turned into information, and no clear information strategy has been formulated. As a result, data collection is haphazard and of dubious quality, making planning dangerously unscientific and cost-effectiveness analysis impossible. Resources have to be devoted to appropriate training of staff.

The research can highlight the key barriers to the functioning of district health management, and allows specific recommendations to be made. The use value of the research for funders is that it pinpoints areas where development assistance can be targeted. The use value for those being researched is that the research provides an analysis of strengths and weaknesses, which can form the start of an action plan to improve managerial effectiveness. Furthermore, it assists in developing methods to achieve targeting of service provisions, especially aimed at the poorest groups.

IMPLICATIONS FOR TRAINING

Returning to the question of how social science research is used in health policy and planning, it is good to remind ourselves of Bulmer's warning that policy-making and the ways social science feeds into it are incredibly complex. Therefore 'there is no unitary account of how policy evolves or how the knowledge-base contributes to its evolution which is wholly satisfactory. As so often, the real world defies easy compartment-alization' (1986, p.5). He goes on to say that as a result of negotiation social science can play an enlightening role.

This book has gone further than enlightenment and has argued for a much closer 'fit' between research, policy and strategy. This depends not only on the concerns that Richardson *et al.* (1990) have expressed relating to defining the purpose and users of research, but fundamentally on how research is understood by both researchers and (potential and actual) users. Two factors are crucial in this respect: first, the way researchers define their enterprise as a flexible one; second, whether policy makers and managers are prepared and able to be reflexive.

To take the first issue, researchers will have to take a dispassionate look at their own approaches, and ask whether their theoretical outlook, their methods and their interactions with users are appropriate to the policy arena. Thus, it does not only involve negotiation on setting an agreed agenda, including formulating the aims and objectives of research, but also being prepared to question established methodologies. This immediately poses questions about the training of social scientists.

It is important for researchers to do good research, that is, research that adheres to quality standards about whether the design is appropriate to the question, the sound application of methodologies and the analysis and presentation of results. At the same time, researchers have to be trained to understand the wider context in which research takes place, taking into account political and managerial imperatives. This does not mean that they compromise scientific objectivity, but that they realize that research is located in the real world, and that they consider the complex reality of implementing research findings. Research is not a detached and cosy activity, it is subject to conflict and negotiation. Thus, researchers have to be trained in the technical aspects of methodology, but also in examining the social contexts in which research takes place. As a result, they have to learn to be creative and adaptive and to analyse the strengths and weaknesses of different methodological paradigms. Importantly, they have to develop their 'people skills', which involve empathy with the questions posed by policy makers and managers, adopting a stance that allows 'transparency' of research, and working in partnership with users.

Research methods courses, as a result, will teach people the technicalities of research, but also the real-life use of research through simulation, case studies and problem-solving. A wider exploration of the varying contexts in which research is carried out has to be an integral part of training in order to illustrate the processes of negotiation surrounding the use of research. The strategic issues of how and why research is used have to be addressed, and similarly the way researchers can influence the dissemination of findings.

It is beyond the scope of this book to map out an agenda for research training, but I have highlighted the importance of a change in attitude on the part of researchers. Research is no longer an activity that can be separate from the real world; it is subject to similar pressures of funding, it has to demonstrate relevance and cost-effectiveness. There is a danger that fundamental research will be squeezed, and thereby an essential contribution to pushing back the boundaries of knowledge. The effects of fundamental research on applied research are considerable in that it informs its theoretical underpinnings. However, the main concern of this book has been with social science research which is intended to be applied in health policy and planning, and a detailed discussion of the place of fundamental research has not been attempted.

The second issue is concerned with the attitudes of policy makers and managers. They will only use research if they are prepared to evaluate their own enterprise, and reflect on past, present or future policies and interventions. This means that training, or at least consciousness-raising, has to be targeted at users. They have to be aware of the potential contribution of research, and equally of its limitations. Research rarely provides instant solutions, but can illuminate options, alternative routes to decision-making or support choices already made. At the same time, policy makers and managers have to accept that research can be an uncomfortable exercise in that its findings are not controllable or predictable precisely because it is designed as a scientific endeavour. They have to learn to cope with this uncertainty.

CONCLUSION

I have argued that social science research has a distinct contribution to make in understanding the complex problems surrounding health and health care. It complements the knowledge which emanates from other disciplines such as epidemiology, economics, geography and so on. I have discussed the way key methodologies can be applied in health services research and inform policy and management. I have concentrated on the one hand on the distinctive strengths and weaknesses of each method; on the other hand the underlying argument has been that research applied in the health context will increasingly be multidisciplinary and multimethod.

Many of the research methodologies described in this book continue to evolve and there is no 'closure' of the discussion on the use and dissemination of research within this field. Much remains to be explored, many methodological developments have to be advanced in order to cope with the infinite complexities of health and health care. At the same time, there is much exciting work already done which is built on a dialogue between researchers, and policy makers and managers, and the case studies demonstrate how the two worlds can come together and formulate solutions to some of the most pressing problems of our time.

References

Advisory Group on Health Technology Assessment (1992) *Effects of Health Technologies; Principles, Practice, Proposals*, Department of Health, Research and Development Division, London.

Alaszewski, A. and Ong, B.N. (eds) (1990) *Normalisation in Practice. Residential Care for Children with a Profound Mental Handicap*, Routledge, London.

Allen, I. (ed) (1990) *Care Managers and Care Management*, Policy Studies Institute supported by the Joseph Rowntree Memorial Trust, London.

Annett, H. and Rifkin, S. (1988) *Improving Urban Health*, World Health Organization, Geneva.

Arber, S. (1991) Class, paid employment and family roles: making sense of structural disadvantage, gender and health status. *Social Science and Medicine*, **32** (4), 425–36.

Ashton, J. (ed) (1992) *Healthy Cities*, Open University Press, Milton Keynes.

Audit Commission (1986) *Making a Reality of Community Care*, HMSO, London.

Ayer, S. and Alaszewski, A. (1986) *Community Care and the Mentally Handicapped: Services for Mothers and Their Mentally Handicapped Children*, Croom Helm, London.

Badger, F., Cameron, E. and Evers, H. (1988) Caseloads under review. *Health Service Journal*, November 10, 1362–63.

Baker, M. (1991) *Research for Marketing*, Macmillan, Basingstoke.

Baldwin, S., Godfrey, C. and Propper, C. (eds) (1990) *Quality of Life. Perspectives and Policies*, Routledge, London.

Banta, D. (1990) *Emerging and Future Health Care Technology and The Nature of the Hospital*, Welsh Health Planning Forum, Cardiff.

Banta, D. (1991) *The Budget is Blind: The Case of Minimally Invasive Therapy in Europe*, TNO Health Research report, Leiden.

Baqwa, J., Kikoito, N., Massaquoi, S., Matsebula, G., Mears, C. (1990) *The Background to and Influencing Factors of the Current Concern about the Alleged Increase of Chest Problems in the Bootle Area*, Liverpool School of Tropical Medicine, Liverpool.

Beardshaw, V. and Towell, D. (1990) *Assessment and Case Management. Implications for the Implementation of 'Caring for People'*, Briefing Paper 10, King's Fund Institute, London.

Bell, C. and Newby, H. (1971) *Community Studies*, Allen and Unwin, London.

Bezold, C. (1991) *On Futures Thinking for Health and Health Care: Trends, Scenarios, Visions and Strategies*, Institute for Alternative Futures, Alexandria, Virginia.

Black, A. (1988) Small is beautiful? *Nursing Times*, **84** (36), 19.

Blaxter, M. (1976) *The Meaning of Disability*, Heinemann, London.

Blaxter, M. (1983) The causes of disease. Women talking. *Social Science and Medicine*, **17** (2), 59–69.

Blaxter, M. (1987) Evidence on inequality in health from a national survey. *The Lancet*, July 4, 30–33.

Blaxter, M. (1990) *Health and Lifestyles*, Routledge, London.

Bowling, A. (1991) *Measuring Health*, Open University Press, Milton Keynes.

Bradshaw, J. (1972) A taxonomy of social need, in *Problems and Progress in Medical Care*, (ed. G.McLachlan), seventh series, Oxford University Press, Oxford, pp.71–82.

Brewer, J. and Hunter, A. (1989) *Multimethod Research. A Synthesis of Styles*, Sage, London.

Bryman, A. (1988) *Quantity and Quality in Social Research*, Unwin Hyman, London.

Buchan, H., Gray, M., Hill, A., Coulter, A. (1990) Needs assessment made simple. *Health Service Journal*, February 15, 240–41.

Bucquet, D. and Curtis, S. (1986) Socio-demographic variation in perceived illness and the use of primary care: the value of community survey data for primary care service planning. *Social Science and Medicine*, **23** (7), 737–44.

Bulmer, M. (1986) Evaluation research and social experimentation, in *Social Science and Social Policy*, (ed. M. Bulmer), Allen and Unwin, London, pp.155–79.

Busfield, J. (1989) Sexism and psychiatry. *Sociology*, **23** (3), 343–64.

Butler, R. (1991) *Designing Organisations. A Decision-making Perspective*, Routledge, London.

Cartwright, A. (1983) *Health Surveys in Practice and Potential: A Critical Review of Their Scope and Methods*, King Edward's Hospital Fund for London, London.

Cartwright, A. and Anderson, R. (1982) *General Practice Revisited: A Second Study of Patients and Their Doctors*, Tavistock, London.

Cartwright, A. and Seale, C. (1990) *A Natural History of a Survey*, King Edward's Hospital Fund for London, London.

Clifford, P. and Holloway, F. (1989) *Evaluating the Closure of Cane Hill Hospital: Protocol for a Collaborative Research Programme with South East Thames RHA*, NUPRD, London.

Comaroff, J. (1976) Communicating information about non-fatal illness: the strategies of a group of General Practitioners. *Sociological Review*, **24** (2), 269–87.

Conway, G. (1988) Editorial. *RRA Notes*, Institute for Environment and Development, **1**, 3.

Cornwell, J. (1984) *Hard Earned Lives: Accounts of Health and Illness from East London*, Tavistock, London.

Cox, B., Blaxter, M., Buckle, A. et al. (1987) *The Health and Lifestyle Survey*, The Health Promotion Trust, London.

Croft, S. and Beresford, P. (1990) *From Paternalism to Participation: Involving People in Social Services*, Open Services Project, London.

Culyer, A. and Wagstaff, A. (1992) *Need, Equity and Equality in Health and Health Care*, Discussion Paper 95, Centre for Health Economics, Health Economics Consortium, University of York, York.

Daatland, S. (1989) *'What are Families For?' On Family Solidarity and Preference for help*, paper presented at the conference on Intergenerational Relations and Equity: Individual and Collective Perspectives, European Behavioral and Social Science Research Section, Dubrovnik.

Daft, R. (1989) *Organisation Theory and Design*, 3rd edn, West Publishing Co., St.Paul, Minn.

Dale, A., Arber, S. and Procter, M. (1988) *Doing Secondary Analysis*, Unwin Hyman, London.

Dalley, G. (1987) Decentralisation: a new way of organising community health services. *Hospital and Health Services Review*, March, 72–4.

Dalley, G. (1988) *Ideologies of Care*, MacMillan, London.

Daly, J. and McDonald, I. (1992) Introduction: the problem as we saw it, in *Researching Health Care: Designs, Dilemmas, Disciplines*, (eds. J. Daly, I. McDonald and E. Willis), Tavistock/Routledge, London, pp.1–12.

Davies, L. (1987) *Quality, Costs and 'An Ordinary Life'*, King's Fund Project Paper No. 67, London.

Dean, T., Rees, M. and Standish, S. (1992) A jigsaw for people. *Health Service Journal*, February 20, 22–23.

Delamothe, T. (1991) Social inequalities in health. *British Medical Journal*, **303**, 1046–50.

Department of Health (1989) *The 1990 General Medical Practitioners' Contract*, HMSO, London.

Department of Health, Department of Social Security, Welsh Office and Scottish Office (1989a) *Caring for People*, CM 849, HSMO, London.

Department of Health, Welsh Office, Scottish Home and Health Department, and Northern Ireland Office (1989b) *Working for Patients*, CM 555, HSMO, London.

Department of Health (1990) *Community Care in the Next Decade and Beyond. Policy Guidance*, HMSO, London.

Department of Health (1991a) *The Health of the Nation: A Consultative Document for Health in England*, CM 1523, HSMO, London.

Department of Health (1991b) *The Patient's Charter*, HMSO, London.

Department of Health (1992) *The Health of the Nation: A Strategy for Health in England*, CM 1986, HSMO, London.

Department of Health and Social Security (1962) *Hospital Plan for England and Wales*, HSMO, London.

Department of Health and Social Security (1975) *Better Services for the Mentally Ill*, CM 6233, HSMO, London.

Devlin, B., Hanham, I., Le Farne, J., Lefever, R., Mantell, B., Freeman, M., (1990) *Medical Care: is it a Common Good?*, IEA Health Unit Paper No.8, London.

Dickenson, J. (1990) *Inspection of Services for People with Physical and Sensory Disabilities 1989/90*, Cheshire Social Services Development Branch, Chester.

Donaldson, C. and Mooney, G. (1991) *Needs Assessment, Priority Setting and Contracts for Health Care: An Economic View*, HERU Discussion Paper 05/91, Aberdeen.

Doyal, L. and Gough, I. (1991) *A Theory of Human Need*, Macmillan, London.

Dun, R. (1989a) *Pictures of Health?*, West Lambeth Health Authority Community Unit, London.

Dun, R. (1989b) *Pictures of Health? Vol.II. Methodology and Research Tools*, West Lambeth Health Authority Community Unit, London.

Farquhar, M., Bowling, A. and Grundy, E. (1992) *Report of the Re-Interviews with Elderly People: Sample Aged 65+ Living at Home in Braintree, Essex*, Department of Public Health, City and Hackney Health Authority.

Farrington, K. (1987) Community management budgeting. *British Journal of Healthcare Computing*, **4** (2), 23–5.

Fazey, C. (1987) *Evaluating Drug Dependency Clinics: Theoretical Frameworks and Methodological Considerations*, Studies of Drug Issues: Report 1, Centre for Urban Studies, Liverpool.

Finch, J. (1986) Age, in *Key Variables in Social Investigation*, (ed. R.Burgess), Routledge and Kegan Paul, London, pp.12–30.

Finch, J. (1987) The vignette technique in survey research. *Sociology*, **21** (1), 105–14.

Finch, J. (1989) *Family Obligations and Social Change*, Polity Press in association with Blackwell, Oxford.

Finch, J. and Groves, D. (eds) (1983) *A Labour of Love*, Routledge and Kegan Paul, London.

Fitzpatrick, R. and Hopkins, A. (1983) Problems in conceptual frameworks of patient satisfaction research: an empirical exploration. *Sociology of Health and Illness*, **5**, 297–311.

Fitzpatrick, R., Newman, S., Archer, R. and Shipley, M. (1991) Social support, disability and depression: a longitudinal study of rheumatoid arthritis. *Social Science and Medicine*, **33**, 605–11.

Flynn, R. (1992) *Structures of Control in Health Management*, Routledge, London.

Freidson, E. (1975) *Profession of Medicine. A Study of the Sociology of Applied Knowledge*, Dodd, Mead and Co., New York.

Freire, P. (1972) *Pedagogy of the Oppressed*, Penguin, Harmondsworth.

Gerhardt, U. (1990) Patients careers in end-stage renal failure. *Social Science and Medicine*, **30**, (11), 1211–24.

Giddens, A. (1989) *Sociology*, Polity Press, Oxford.

Glaser, B. and Strauss, A. (1967) The *Discovery of Grounded Theory: Strategies for Qualitative Research*, Aldine Publishing Co., Chicago.

Glendinning, C. (1986) *A Single Door: Social Work with the Families of Disabled Children*, Allen and Unwin, London.

Goffman, E. (1961) *Asylums. Essays in the Social Situation of Mental Patients and Other Inmates*, Doubleday, New York.

Goldberg, D. and Hillier, V. (1979) A scaled version of the General Health Questionnaire. *Psychological Medicine*, **9**, 139–45.

Green, H. (1988) *Informal Carers: a Study*, OPCS, HSMO, London.

Griffiths, Sir Roy. (1988) *Community Care: An Agenda for Action*, A report to the Secretary of State for Social Services, HSMO, London.

Hakim, C. (1987) *Research Design*, Allen and Unwin, London.

Halfpenny, P. (1979) The analysis of qualitative data. *Sociological Review*, **27** (4), 799–827.

Hammersley, M. (1990) What's wrong with ethnography? The myth of theoretical description. *Sociology*, **24** (4), 597–616.

Hammersley, M. (1992) *What's Wrong with Ethnography?*, Routledge, London.

Hammersley, M. and Atkinson, P. (1983) *Ethnography: Principles in Practice*, Tavistock, London.

Harpurhey Resettlement Project (1987) *'Getting to Know You' Project*, Manchester.

Harrison, S., Hunter, D. and Pollitt, C. (1990) *The Dynamics of British Health Policy*, Unwin Hyman, London.

Hawker, M. (1989) Consumer participation as community development: action in an ambiguous context. *Community Development Journal*, **24** (4), October, 283–91.

Hellevik, O. (1984) *Introduction to Causal Analysis*, Allen and Unwin, London.

Helman, C. (1990) *Culture, Health and Illness*, 2nd edn, Wright, London.

Herzlich, C. (1973) *Health and Illness*, Academic Press, London.

Higginson, I., Wade, A., McCarthy, M. (1990) Palliative care: views of patients and their families. *British Medical Journal*, **301**, 277–81.

Hillery, G. (1955) Definitions of community: areas of agreement. *Rural Sociology*, **80**, 2, 111–23.

Hirst, M. (1990) Multidimensional representation of disablement: a qualitative approach, in *Quality of Life: Perspectives and Policies*, (eds. S. Baldwin, C. Godfrey and C. Propper), Routledge, London, pp.72–83.

Hoinville, G., Jowell, R. et al., (1977) *Survey Research Practice*, Heinemann, London.

Holmes, C. (1989) Health care and the quality of life: a review. *Journal of Advanced Nursing*, **14**, 833–9.

Horn, J. (1969) *Away with all Pests*, Monthly Review Press, New York.

Hudson, B. (1990) Yes, but will it work? *Health Service Journal*, February 1, 169–70.

Hugman, R. (1991) *Power in Caring Professions*, Macmillan, Basingstoke.

Humphris, G. and Ong, B. N. *et al.* (1990) *Health and Lifestyle: a Survey in South Sefton*, South Sefton Health Authority, Liverpool.

Hunt, S., McKenna, S. and McEwan, J. (1986) *Measuring Health Status*, Croom Helm, London.

Hunter, D. (1990a) Beware: species at risk. *Health Service Journal*, May 3, 673.

Hunter, D. (1990b) Organising and managing health care: a challenge for medical sociology, in *Readings in Medical Sociology* (eds. S. Cunningham-Burley and N. McKeganey), Tavistock/Routledge, London, pp.213–36.

Hunter, D. (1991) Managing medicine: a response to the 'crisis'. *Social Science and Medicine*, **32** (4), 441–9.

Hyman, H. (1955) *Survey Design and Analysis*, Free Press, Glencoe, Illinois.

Illsley, R. (1980) *Professional or Public Health?*, Nuffield Provincial Hospitals Trust, London.

Illsley, R. and Baker, D. (1991) Contextual variations in the meaning of health inequality. *Social Science and Medicine*, **32** (4), 359–65.

Illsley, R. and Le Grand, J. (1987) The measurement of inequality in health, in *Health and Economics*, (ed. A.Williams), Macmillan, Basingstoke, pp.12–36.

Ingleby, D. (1983) The social construction of mental illness, in *The problem of Medical Knowledge: Examining the Social Construction of Medicine* (eds. A. Treacher and P. Wright), Edinburgh University Press, Edinburgh, pp.123–43.

Isabella, L. (1990) Evolving interpretations as a change unfolds: how managers construe key organisational events. *Academy of Management Journal*, **33** (1), 7–41.

Jacobson, B., Smith, A. and Whitehead, M. (1991) *The Nation's Health. A Strategy for the 1990s*. King Edward's Hospital Fund for London, London.

Jarman, B. (1983) Identification of underprivileged areas. *British Medical Journal*, **286**, 1705–9.

Jefferys, M. (1991) The agenda for sociological health policy research for the 1990s, in *The Sociology of the Health Service*, (eds. J. Gabe, M. Calnan and M. Bury), Routledge, London, pp.222–32.

Jefferys, M. and Thane, P. (1989) Introduction: an ageing society and ageing people, in *Growing Old in the Twentieth Century*, (ed. M. Jefferys), Routledge, London, pp.1–18.

Kay, A. and Legg, C. (1986) *Discharged to the community. A Review of Housing and Support in London for People Leaving Psychiatric Care*, Good Practices in Mental Health, London.

Kendall, A. and Dodson, G. (1990) Researching the Croxteth Park Project. The costs and benefits to the Agency, in *Normalisation in Practice*, (eds. A. Alaszewski and B.N. Ong), Routledge, London, pp.48–55.

Kerlinger, F. (1973) *Foundations of Behavioural Research*, 2nd edn., Holt, Rinehart and Winston, New York.

Kirkham, M. (1986) A feminist perspective in midwifery, in *Feminist Practice in Women's Health Care*, (ed. C. Webb), J. Wiley and Sons, Chichester, pp.35–50.

Klein, L. (1990) *Two Nations? The Annual Report on the Health of the Population in South Sefton, 1989/90*, South Sefton (Merseyside) Health Authority, Liverpool.

Klein, R. (1991) Making sense of inequalities: a response to Peter Townsend. International Journal of Health Services, **21** (1), 175–81.

Kuhn, T. (1970) *The Structure of Scientific Revolutions*, 2nd edn., University of Chicago Press, Chicago.

Kuipers, L. (1987) Research in expressed emotion. *Social Psychiatry*, **22**, 216–20.

Lalonde, M. (1974) *A New Perspective on the Health of Canadians*, Government of Canada, Ottawa.

Land, H. (1991) Time to care, in *Women's Issues in Social Policy*, (eds. M. MacLean and D. Groves), Routledge, London, pp.7–19.

Leedham, I. and Wistow, G. (1992) *Community Care and General Practitioners*, Nuffield Institute for Health Services Studies, Leeds.

Lees, R. and Smith, H. (eds) (1977) *Action Research and Community Development*, Routledge and Kegan Paul, London.

Levine, A. (1984) A model for health projections using knowledgeable informants. *World Health Statistics Quarterly*, **37**, 306–13.

Limb, M. (1992) The poverty of theory. *Health Service Journal*, July 16, 13.

Lincoln, Y. and Guba, E. (1985) *Naturalistic Inquiry*, Sage, Beverley Hills.

Locker, D. (1981) *Symptoms and Illness*, Tavistock, London.

Locker, D. and Dunt, D. (1979) Theoretical and methodological issues in sociological studies of consumer satisfaction. *Social Science and Medicine*, **12**, 283–92.

Lundberg, G., Schrag, A. and Larsen, O. (1958) *Sociology*, Harper and Row, New York.

Lyons Morris, L., Taylor Fitz-Gibbon, C. and Freeman, M. (1987) *How to Communicate Evaluation Findings*, Sage, Newbury Park.

Marmot, M. and McDowall, M. (1986) Mortality decline and widening social inequalities. *The Lancet*, **II** (8501), 274–6.

Marsden, D. and Oakley, P. (1991) Future issues and perspectives in the evaluation of social development. *Community Development Journal*, **26** (4), 314–28.

Marsh, C. (1982) *The Survey Method: the Contribution of Surveys to Sociological Explanation*, Allen and Unwin, London.

Martin, J., Meltzer, H. and Elliot, D. (1988) *The Prevalence of Disability Among Adults*, OPCS Surveys of Disability in Great Britain, Report 1, OPCS, HMSO, London.

Maxwell, R. (1984) Quality assessment in health. *British Medical Journal*, **288**, 1470–72.

Mays, N. (in press) The way of the new, in *Dilemmas in Health Care*, (eds. B. Davey and J. Popay), Open University Press, Buckingham.

Mays, N., Petrukevich, A. and Snowdon, C. (1990) Patients' quality of life following extra-corporeal shockwave lithotripsy and percutaneous nephrolithotomy for renal calculi. *International Journal for Technology Assessment in Health Care*, **6**, 633–42.

McDonald, R. and Blizard, R. (1988) Quality assurance of outcome in mental health care: a model for routine use in clinical settings. *Health Trends*, **20**, 111–4.

McIntosh, J. (1977) *Communications and Awareness in a Cancer Ward*, Croom Helm, London.

McIver, S. (1991) *An Introduction to Obtaining the Views of Users of Health Services*, King's Fund Centre, London.

McKee, M. (1991) Health services in central and eastern Europe: past problems and future prospects. *Journal of Epidemiology and Community Health*, 85–90.

McKenzie, M., Critchley, M. and Mercer, N. (1990) *Thatto Heath: a Rapid Appraisal survey*, St. Helens.

Megone, C. (1990) The quality of life. Starting from Aristotle, in *Quality of life: Perspectives and Policies*, (eds. S. Baldwin, C. Godfrey and C. Propper), Routledge, London, pp.28–39.

MIND (1989–90), *'People First' Questionnaire, 1989–1990*, MIND, London.

Mintzberg, H. and Waters, J. (1990) Does decision get in the way? *Organization Studies*, **11**, 1, 1–6.

Mitchell, J., Clyde (1983) Case and situation analysis. *Sociological Review*, **31**, 187–211.

Morris, J. (1990) Inequalities in health: ten years, and little further on. *British Medical Journal*, **301**, 491–3.

Moser, C. and Kalton, G. (1971) *Survey Methods in Social Investigation*, 2nd edn, Heinemann, London.

National Schizophrenia Fellowship (1985) *Cart Before the Horse?* The correspondence between the Chairman of the NSF and the Minister for Health, February 1984 to July 1985, National Schizophrenia Fellowship, London.

Nichter, M. (1984) Project community diagnosis: participatory research as a first step towards community involvement in primary health care. *Social Science and Medicine*, **19** (3), 237–52.

Nyamwaya, D. (1987) A case study of the interaction between indigenous and western medicine among the Pokot of Kenya. *Social Science and Medicine*, **25** (12), 1277–87.

Oakley, A. (1981a) *Subject Women*, Martin Robertson, Oxford.

Oakley, A. (1981b) Interviewing women: a contradiction in terms, in *Doing Feminist Research*, (ed. H.Roberts), Routledge and Kegan Paul, London, pp.30–61.

O'Brien, J. and Tyne, A. (1981) *The Principle of Normalisation: a Foundation for Effective Services*, CMH, London.

Ong, B. N. (1989) Research from within: blurring boundaries and developing new models. *Sociological Review*, **37** (3), 505–17.

Ong, B. N. (1991) Researching needs in District Nursing. *Journal of Advanced Nursing*, **16**, 638–47.

Ong, B. N. (1993) The development of Minimally Invasive Therapy in the United Kingdom. *Health Policy*, **23**, 83–95.

Ong, B. N. and Humphris, G. (1990) Partners in need. *Health Service Journal*, July 5, 1002–3.

Ong, B. N., Humphris, G., Annett, H. and Rifkin, S. (1991) Rapid Appraisal in an urban setting; an example from the developed world. *Social Science and Medicine*, **32** (8), 909–15.

Ong, B. N. and Shiels, C. (1991) *Understanding User Need and Preference: Exploring New Methodologies*, EHMA Conference, Toledo.

Orem, D. (1980) *Nursing: Concepts of Practice*, McGraw Hill, New York.

Pahl, R. (1984) *Divisions of Labour*, Blackwell, Oxford.

Parker, G. (1990) *With Due Care and Attention*, Family Policy Studies Centre, London.

Patmore, C. (1989) Is patient power coming to Britain? *Community Psychiatry*, October, 34–5.

Paton, C. and Bach, S. (1990) *Case Studies in Health Policy and Management*, Nuffield Provincial Hospitals Trust, London.

Paton, C., Ong, B. N. and Shiels, C. (in progress) *Project Orange. Resource Management Project: Care of the Elderly*, Crewe Health Authority and Cheshire Family Health Service Authority.

Patrick, D. and Peach, H. (eds) (1989) *Disablement in the Community*, Oxford Medical Publications, Oxford University Press, Oxford.

Peach, H. and Patrick, D. (1989) A strategy for community provision, in *Disablement in the Community*, (eds. D. Patrick and H. Peach), Oxford Medical Publications, Oxford University Press, Oxford, pp.197–211.

Peckham, M. (1991) *Research for Health. A Research and Development Strategy for the NHS*, Department of Health, Research and Development Division, London.

Personal Social Services Research Unit (1987) *Care in the Community*, University of Kent, Canterbury.

Pettigrew, A. (1990) Studying strategic choice and strategic change: a comment on Mintzberg and Waters 'Does decision get in the way?'. *Organization Studies*, **11** (1), 1–16.

Pettigrew, A., Ferlie, E. and McKee, L. (1992) *Shaping Strategic Change*, Sage, London.

Pettigrew, A., McKee, L and Ferlie, E. (1988) Understanding change in the NHS. *Public Administration*, **66** (3), 297–317.

Popay, J., Williams, G., Ong, B. N. and Edwards, J. (1992) *Involving Local People in the NHS: A Guide to the Role of Qualitative Research*, Department of Health, London.

Porter, M. and MacIntyre, S. (1984) What is, must be best: a research note on conservative or deferential responses to antenatal provision. *Social Science and Medicine*, **19** (11), 1197–200.

Pritchard, A. (ed) (1988) *Cancer nursing – a Revolution in Care*, Proceedings of the Fifth International Conference on cancer nursing, Macmillan, Basingstoke.

Radical Statistics Group (1991) Missing: a strategy for health of the nation. *British Medical Journal*, **303**, 299–302.

Ramon, S. (ed) (1987) *Psychiatry in Transition*, Zed Books, London.

Raphael, W. (1977) *Patients and Their Hospitals*, King Edward's Hospital Fund for London, London.

Rathwell, T. (1992) Pursuing Health for All in Britain – an assessment. *Social Science and Medicine*, **34** (2), 169–82.

Research Unit in Health and Behavioural Change (1989) *Changing the Public Health*, J. Wiley and Sons, Chichester.

Renfrew, M. and McCandlish, R. (1992) With women: new steps in research in midwifery, in *Women's health matters*, (ed. H. Roberts), Routledge, London, pp.81–98.

Richardson, A., Jackson, C. and Sykes, W. (1990) *Taking Research Seriously*, HMS, London.

Rifkin, S., Muller, F. and Bichmann, W. (1988) Primary Health Care: on measuring participation. *Social Science and Medicine*, **26** (9), 931–40.

Riley, M. White (1963) *Sociological Research I. A Case Approach*, Harcourt, Brace and World Inc., New York.

Roberts, J. (1992) *Evolving Interpretations of Change. How Managers Construe Key Issues in Developing New Roles*, Unpublished MBA. Thesis, Keele University, Keele.

Roper, N., Logan, W. and Tierney, A. (1980) *The Elements of Nursing*, Churchill Livingstone, Edinburgh.

Roscam Abbing, E. (1992) *The Future of Public Health: a Scenario Study*, Scenario report commissioned by the Steering Committee on Future Health Scenarios, Kluwer Academic Publishers, Dordrecht, London.

Roy, C. and Roberts, S. (1981) *Theory Construction in Nursing: an Adaptation Model*, Prentice Hall, New Jersey.

Salmen, L. (1987) *Listen to People*, Oxford University Press, Oxford.

Schoon, N. (1992) Families blame coaldust for asthma among their children. *The Independent*, February 5, 8.

Scott-Samuel, A. (1986) Social inequalities in health: back on the agenda. *The Lancet*, 1, 1084–5.

Sculpher, M. and Buxton, M. (1991) *Report of Phase I of the Medical Laser Technology Assessment*, HERG Research Report No.9, Brunel University, Uxbridge.

Shiell, A. and Wright, K. (1990) The economic costs, in *Normalisation in Practice* (eds. A. Alaszewski and B.N. Ong), Routledge, London, pp.249–66.

Shiels, C. (1991) *Regional Specialties Project: Factors Influencing Choice of Methodology*, Centre for Health Planning and Management, Keele University, Keele.

Shiels, C. (1992a) *Regional Specialties Questionnaire: Methodology, Validity and Reliability*, Centre for Health Planning and Management, Keele University, Keele.

Shiels, C. (1992b) *Project Orange: Survey of Health Needs of the Elderly*, Centre for Health Planning and Management, Keele University, Keele.

Sidel, R. and Sidel, V. (1983) *The Health of China*, Zed Books, London.

Small, N. (1989) *Politics and Planning in the National Health Service*, Open University Press, Milton Keynes.

Smith, G. and Cantley, C. (1985) *Assessing Health Care*, Open University Press, Milton Keynes.

Smith, R. (1987) *Unemployment and Health*, Oxford University Press, Oxford.

Snee, K. (ed) (1991) *Dallam on Health*, Warrington.

Spradley, J. (1980) *Participant Observation*, Holt, Rinehart and Winston, New York.

St Leger, A., Schnieden, H. and Walsworth-Bell, J. (1992) *Evaluating Health Services' Effectiveness*, Open University Press, Milton Keynes.

Stacey, M. (1988) *The Sociology of Health and Healing*, Unwin Hyman, London.

Stacey, M. (1991) Medical Sociology and Health Policy: An Historical Overview, *The Sociology of the Health Service*, (eds. J. Gabe, M. Calnan and M. Bury), Routledge, London, pp.11–35.

Stanley, L (1990) Doing ethnography, writing ethnography: a comment on Hammersley. *Sociology*, 24 (4), 617–28.

Stanley, L. and Wise, S. (1983) *Breaking Out: Feminist Consciousness and Feminist Research*, Routledge and Kegan Paul, London.

Steering Group on Future Health Scenarios. (1991) *Chronic Diseases in the Year 2005. Vol.1. Scenarios on Diabetus Mellitus, 1990–2005*, Kluwer Academic Publishers, Dordrecht.

Stevens, A. and Gabbay, J. (1991) Needs assessment needs assessment. *Health Trends*, 23 (1), 20–3.

Stewart-Brown, S. and Protheroe, D. (1988) Evaluation in community development. *Health Education Journal*, 47 (4), 156–61.

Stimson, G. and Webb, B. (1975) *Going to See the Doctor*, Routledge and Kegan Paul, London.

Stocking, B. (1984) *Initiative and Inertia; Case Studies in the NHS*, Nuffield Provincial Hospitals Trust, London.

Strauss, A., Schatzman, L., Ehrlich, D., Bucher, R., Sabshin, M. (1963) The hospital and its negotiated order, in *The Hospital in Modern Society*, (ed. E.Freidson), Collier-Macmillan, London, pp.147–69.

Strong, P. (1979) *The Ceremonial Order of the Clinic*, Routledge and Kegan Paul, London.

Strong, P. and Robinson, J. (1990) *The NHS under New Management*, Open University Press, Milton Keynes.

Thane, P. (1989) Old age: burden or benefit?, in *The Changing Population of Britain*, (ed. H. Joshi), Basil Blackwell, Oxford, pp.56–71.

Thompson, A. (1983) *The Measurement of Patients' Perception of the Quality of Hospital Care*, UMIST, Manchester.

Thunhurst, C. (1985) *Poverty and Health in the City of Sheffield*, Environmental Health Department, Sheffield City Council, Sheffield.

Tomlinson, D. (1991) *Utopia, Community Care and the Retreat from the Asylums*, Open University Press, Milton Keynes.

Torkington, P. (1991) *Black Health: a Political Issue*, Catholic Association for Racial Justice and Liverpool Institute of Higher Education, Liverpool.

Townsend, P. (1990) Widening inequalities of health in Britain: a rejoinder to Rudolph Klein. *International Journal of Health Services*, **20** (3), 363–72.

Townsend, P. (1991) Evading the issue of widening inequalities of health in Britain: a reply to Rudolph Klein. *International Journal of Health Services*, **21** (1), 183–9.

Townsend, P and Davidson, N. (1982) *Inequalities in Health: the Black Report*, Penguin, Harmondsworth.

Townsend, P., Phillimore, P. and Beattie, A. (1988) *Health and Deprivation. Inequality and the North*, Croom Helm, London.

Twigg, J., and Atkin, K. (1990) *Informal Care and the Process of Service Delivery*, paper delivered at the Medical Sociology Conference, Edinburgh, September 15.

Twigg, J., Atkin, K. and Perring, C. (1990) *Carers and Services. A Review of Research*, HMSO, London.

Varkevisser, C., Nuyens, Y. and Stott, G. (1990) *Health Systems Research – Does It Make a Difference? The Joint WHO/DGIS/RTI Project on Health Systems Research for the Southern Africa Region*, World Health Organization, Geneva.

de Vaus, D. (1990) *Surveys in Social Research*, 2nd edn. Unwin Hyman, London.

Vaux, A., Riedel, S. and Stewart, D. (1987) Modes of social support: the Social Support Behaviour (SS-B) scale. *American Journal of Community Psychology*, **15**, 209–33.

Waitzkin, H. and Stoeckle, D. (1972) The communication of information about illness: clinical, sociological and methodological considerations. *Advances in Psychosomatic Medicine*, **8**, 180–215.

Welsh Office (1989a) *Strategic Intent and Direction for the NHS in Wales*, NHS Directorate, Welsh Health Planning Forum.

Welsh Office (1989b) *Local Strategies for Health: A New Approach to Strategic Planning*, NHS Directorate, Welsh Health Planning Forum.

Wenger, G.C. (1987) *The Research Relationship. Practice and Politics in Social Policy Research*, Allen and Unwin, London.

Wenger, G.C. (1989) Support networks in old age: constructing a typology, in *Growing Old in the Twentieth Century*, (ed. M. Jefferys), Routledge, London, pp.166–85.

Whitehead, M. (1987) *The Health Divide: Inequalities in Health in the 1980s*, Health Education Authority, London.

Whyte, W, Foote. (1984) Participant observation: rationale and roles, in *Learning from the Field*, (ed. W. Foote Whyte), Sage, Beverly Hills, pp.23–34.

Wiggins, D. and Dermen, S. (1987) Needs, need and needing. *Journal of Medical Ethics*, **13** (2), 62–8.

Wilkin, D., Hallam, L. and Doggatt, M-A. (1992) *Measures of Need and Outcome in Primary Care*, Oxford Medical Publications, Oxford.

Wilkin, D., Hallam, L., Leavey, R. and Metcalfe, D. (1987) *Anatomy of Urban General Practice*, Tavistock, London.

Williams, A. (1985) Economics of coronary artery bypass grafting. *British Medical Journal*, **291**, 326–9.

Williams, A. (1987) Measuring quality of life: a comment. *Sociology*, **21** (4), 565–6.

Williams, S. and Allen, I. (1989) *Health Care for Single Homeless People*, Policy Studies Institute, London.

Wolfensberger, W. (1983) Social role valorisation: a proposed new term for the principle of normalisation. *Mental Retardation*, **21** (6), 234–9.

World Health Organization (1980) *International Classification of Impairment, Disabilities and Handicaps*, World Health Organization, Geneva.

World Health Organization (1981) *Global Strategy for Health for All by the Year 2000*, World Health Organization, Geneva.

World Health Organization (1985) *Targets for Health for All 2000*, WHO Regional Office for Europe, Copenhagen.

World Health Organization Programme on Health Systems Research and Development (1988) *Health Systems Research in Action. Case studies from Botswana, Colombia, Egypt, Indonesia, Malaysia, the Netherlands, Norway and the United States of America*, World Health Organization, Geneva.

Yin, R. (1984) *Case Study Research: Design and Method*, Sage, Beverley Hills.

Index